THE
PHOENIX DIARIES

A Journey of Pain, Power, and Purpose

by Dr. Nicole Schtupak

Edited by Lil Barcaski

Published by: GWN Publishing
www.GWNPublishing.com

Cover Design: Kristina Conatser

ISBN: 978-1-965971-40-6

DEDICATION

I dedicate this book to anyone who has ever felt lost, out of place, broken, or unsure of the path ahead — whether for a fleeting moment or a lifetime.

Step beyond your comfort zone.

Trust in your ability to achieve what you set your mind to.

Shift your perspective — it is worth it. Every time.

You are not alone.

We are all walking this journey together.

You are capable. You are worthy.

Rise as many times as it takes.

After all... You are the Phoenix!

TABLE OF CONTENTS

Pain

CHAPTER 1

THE TRUTH WILL SET THINGS ON FIRE

The embers of who I once was, the truth of my being rose, unexpected, unyielding, and entirely my own. The flames that I thought would destroy me instead stripped me bare, revealing the woman I was always meant to be. Reflecting, the moment that was the catalyst to who I was occurred when I was about six to seven years old. I was doing my chores, cleaning the house for my mom, when I noticed a bunch of papers on the floor of a closet next to one of those old accordion folders people used to store paperwork in. Among the documents on the floor near the accordion folder, one had my biological father's name on it and the name of a woman that I'd never heard of or seen before. I didn't understand much of what that paper was other than it seemed to be some sort of legal thing. My almost seven-year-old brain concluded that made sense to me in the moment. My father must have had an affair with this woman, and there was some sort of lawsuit or something. I remember thinking, maybe this was why my parents had recently divorced.

I'll never forget the moment I came across this document. Angry and defending my mother, I called my dad immediately. He worked at King Toyota as a mechanic at the time. He may have been a shitty father, but I have to admit, he is a phenomenal mechanic and a pretty intelligent person. The divorce was very recent, so when I got him on the phone, I went into accusation mode. "Now I know why Mom left you. It's because you cheated on her." Confused, he asked why I would think that. I informed him of the paper I had found. He replied, "You have that all wrong. I didn't cheat on your mother. Put the paper back; it has nothing to do with you." I didn't believe him, but I didn't have much choice. I didn't want to upset my mom and was unsure if they would discuss the phone call, so I dropped the subject and put the papers in the folder and back where I found them.

Not too long after the divorce, my mom, Andrea, met a wonderful man named Steven, and they started dating. At first, I wasn't too happy about it because I held the dim hope that mom and dad would reunite. Over time, I realized that Steven was so good to my mother, my younger sister, and me. Eventually, I warmed up to the idea of him becoming our stepfather. It is my firm belief that the universe places people in our lives for a reason. In his case, it was to save us. Mom was working three jobs when she and dad divorced to make ends meet. Waiting tables at Wags, working at the Broward County Courthouse traffic division, and in real estate. Despite my young age at the time, after they divorced and seeing how hard mom was working, I felt a strong urge to "grow up" and help as much as I could. She worked long hours to ensure that my sister and I were never without. To this day, I am not sure she truly understands how much I respect, love, and appreciate her. Through it all, she has been my rock. My soulmate. She and Steven saved me in ways they will never understand.

Eventually, Mom and Steven got married, I must have been around eight to nine years old at the time, and we moved to his villa in Pompano. While this was several months after finding that document, the paper from the closet still loomed in the back of my mind. I dismissed it because finally things at home were stable and good. I used to be so sad I shaved off my eyebrows and pulled out my eyelashes when I was about ten years old. I did this so that no one could see the expressions on my face because I did not know how to process all the anxiety and sadness. In my mind, I was "hiding in plain sight." I tried to hide how I was feeling from everyone. But now, things were finally settling down. So I continually rejected any idea of what that paper really was.

I was probably around 11 years old when one afternoon, I came home from school to find my biological father, whom I will refer to as "T," my maternal grandmother, Arlene, my mother, Andrea, and my stepdad, Steven, all in the house, seemingly waiting for me to get there. I was very confused to see them all together and instantly thought *something bad must have happened.* I remember walking in and saying to myself, *What the heck is this*? This was not a sight you would normally see, having all of them under one roof at the same time.

"Nicole, honey, we have something important to tell you," Mom began. "We think you're old enough to know the truth, and we want it to come from us." I couldn't imagine what she would be referring to. Everyone I loved was in the room, so it wasn't likely that someone died. Maybe one of them was sick? They proceeded to tell me that the woman I had always thought to be my mother, Andrea, was not my biological mom. My biological donor's name was Hildagunde, the same name that was on that paper in the folder I had found in the closet over a year prior. I refer to her as my biological donor because in my mind, even more so nowadays, the title "mom" is earned regardless of if you gave birth to the child or not. To me, it is a term of endearment not just a label. Someone who has been there through it all. Standing by and weathering out the storms. Not just when it's all rainbows and unicorns.

My mom, grandma, and biological father explained that was one of the names she went by. It was not clear what her real name was. "T" said that even he was not sure. According to him, he never met her parents and assumed that she was adopted or estranged from her family. Honestly, I have always felt that to be weird. How do you involve yourself with someone so much so to have a child with them and never know their family, their upbringing, etc.? "T" has always been very tight-lipped on details of her. Assume it is from wanting to "protect" me, but c'mon, let's look at this. How much worse could the details of her be? I'm sure he has his reasons, and surrounding details about her, but I don't think I'll ever really know. He always deferred to them "being young," and he did not ask questions. As a result, he said other names she went by were Elizabeth Addison and Elizabeth Perkins, so any variation of those names could be true. I was told that "T" and this woman met when they were very young while he was in the army. Supposedly, my bio-donor was a drug addict and was in her own *Lost World*. My father knew those things about her, but even so, one thing led to another. They fell in love. They got married. They had me.

It is well known that my father has a real issue with telling the truth, so I have no idea if she was on drugs when she got pregnant with me, but according to him, supposedly, none of that kind of behavior was going on at that point. He told me that she was excited to have me. They married when he was 19 and she was 18. According to him, he was in the army, and she was an exotic dancer. After finding out she was pregnant with me, she quit doing drugs, or so he thought. Who knows? They had their issues, but when I was born, I was a healthy baby. Mom, "T," and Grandma Arlene said my biological donor was troubled, suffering from drug abuse and possible mental disorders, and because of this, she wasn't able to take care of a baby. During the conversation, I could tell they tried to downplay things. "She loved you and wanted you, but she had problems," they said. They left out a lot in that first talk.

These many years later, my mom still talks about how she struggled with when and how to tell me the truth. She did bring me to counseling before and after finding out. They were trying to find the best way to tell me. As a group, they realized that it would be better to tell me before I got into my rebellious teen years and found out somehow on my own, especially after finding that document.

When I found out Andrea was not my biological mother, it broke me at first. If you think about it, how does an 11-year-old process that? Everything was set ablaze. However, looking back, I'm glad that I found out then, because all of the lashing out that followed, all of the pain, despite every dark path, I got through it, thank God. Mom used to tell me that "God made a mistake and corrected it by giving me to her and Steven." But when they sat me down that day, I quietly sat there listening, feeling so many emotions. I've told my mom that I do not know where I would be if it weren't for her, and on the other hand, at the time I remember thinking, *What did I do wrong? Why are they lying to me? Why didn't my biological donor and father love me? Why would she leave me? If she loved me as they said she did, why did she give me away? Why are they saying this? Am I so unlovable?*

I couldn't put it all together. When they were done explaining what had happened and who they all were in reality, I stood up, feeling all kinds of emotions, went upstairs, and slammed the door to my bedroom so loud and so hard that it cracked the doorframe from the surge of emotions. Grandma Arlene came up and tried to comfort me. She said that it was because she loved me that she gave me up. Still, despite her attempt, I felt alone. Sad. Unlovable. Discarded.

Years later, I found papers from the hospital where I was born. A new reality hit. My family didn't tell me the whole story. Now, I was older, and I made them tell me everything about what really happened. I needed to know. I needed to know who I really was. So, I kept pushing. What a story it turned out to be.

DAD JOINS THE CIRCUS

Less than six months after I was born, my father decided to call it quits with my birth mother. He found out that she had cheated on him and couldn't handle it, so he left. He took off and literally joined the circus. Every time I think about that statement, it makes me laugh. But it is true. Barnum and Bailey hired him to work as a mechanic, and he travelled with them.

I was born in Orlando, and my dad's sister, we will call her "CeCe," and "T's" mother, Karlene, lived somewhere in the area. Before leaving with the circus, he took me to my aunt's house and dropped me off. She had me for a "little while" when my "biological donor," as I prefer to refer to her, came and picked me up from CeCe's. It's entirely unclear if my aunt "CeCe" knew all the details about her drug abuse, infidelity, etc., but according to what my biological father stated, she did not have a choice but to hand me back to her. From there, Hildegunde took me back home with her, taking me back to the home she and "T" had been living in.

Soon after, unclear of the exact days, Hildegunde decided to run off and left me in a house alone. At that point, I was less than six months old. Thank God, a neighbor heard a baby's cries coming from the house. Noting that the neighbor hadn't seen anyone coming or going to the place for at least three days, the neighbor assumed an infant was left alone in a home for three days and needed help. If there was anyone in the world that I wished I could meet, it would be that neighbor who called HRS (now known as DFS, Department of Family Services) after hearing me cry and seeing no one for days. I would love to meet either them or one of their family members because ultimately that person saved my life. My grandma, Arlene, told me, "She took everything in the house except for you. She supposedly took off with her drug buddies." It is not known exactly where she went or what she was thinking, leaving me in the house alone. No supervision. Not fed or changed. As an infant. What is known is that she was using again and may not have been in the right state of mind.

DFS took me directly to a local hospital. I was malnourished, dehydrated, and not expected to live. I was not fed for at least three days. As an infant, I spent 28 days in the PICU (pediatric ICU), and they designated me, *failure to thrive*. Grandma Arlene explained that I went into cardiac arrest a few times from severe electrolyte abnormalities, and I was critically ill. The details surrounding my admission to the hospital still have some gaps, but DFS somehow contacted my Aunt "CeCe" to let her know that I was in the hospital. Both of my parents abandoned me, and that left her as my next of kin. It was up to her to make all the decisions. According to medical records and Grandma Arlene, because I was so sick, the decision was made that if something like cardiac arrest happened again, and I was not responding to treatments, to just let me go. Over the 28 days in the ICU, not much seemed to be helping me get better. I was depressed, not eating, and not improving. I had IVs in my neck, and each time I look in the mirror, I am reminded of this PICU stay. At the time, the decision was made that if I had gone into distress again, they weren't going to do anything.

Throughout my life, anytime I would feel sad, hopeless, defeated because of life, my grandmother Arlene would say, "Nikki, you've been a fighter since the beginning. You have a purpose. When all seemed as if it was over on the 28th day, you came back. Against the odds, you fought and came back. You're a miracle child. You were meant to be with us." She has since passed away due to complications related to pancreatic cancer. She was always one of my strongest advocates. She would always try to lift my spirits when I felt down. Especially after the divorce and my being informed of the adoption, she would say, "Nikki, you were meant to be with us, even though you were not born into the family, it was meant to be. We have the same eyes. You are meant to be ours." I have hazel green eyes, and she did too. That was her thing. She always would remind me of my strength, resilience, and how we had the same color eyes. She was right; it did make me feel better. Since her passing, I have wished to hear those words again. I miss her voice, and she always made me smile.

Many of the details regarding my biological donor and what she knew of my admission to the ICU and critical status are not known.

Despite many attempts to ask my Aunt "CeCe" and paternal grandmother, Karlene, it was tightly kept under wraps. When I asked "T," he would say that he was not around and that my aunt and paternal grandmother knew. But I never received straight answers. What I do know is that my biological donor showed up at the hospital. When the initial conversation about my adoption came out, I learned that she was presumed to be dead. But it is not entirely clear. My father used to say that she was killed in a car accident when she went to the store. Another story from him was that she was shot while going to the store. I had also been told that she was so "gone" from all the drugs she did. So, in all honesty, I have no idea what really happened to her. I remember thinking that I could stand next to her in line at the grocery store and would never know. "T" also said that his mother kept a lot from him. Perhaps that is true, but I never understood why that would be. According to him, Karlene had stayed in contact with my biological donor and knew how to reach her for quite some time. I always felt that to be odd. Especially keeping all the details from me. When I was hospitalized from neglect and failure to thrive, Karlene alerted her to what was happening. The hospital staff and DFS had a lot of questions for Hildegunde. I guess that must have scared her off, and she bolted. From what I know, she never showed up again. I can't understand why she did not get arrested, but a police officer we know said that even up to the late 1980s, child abandonment was a misdemeanor, not much worse than stealing a pack of gum from a convenience store. So, she "got away" with what she did to me, and no one seems to have ever heard from her again, including me. On that 28th day after cardiac arrest from severe electrolyte abnormalities, I was "reborn." Arlene said, "When all was lost and there was not going to be anymore intervention, you came back and from there, you began responding to treatments. You got stronger. You are a fighter, Nikki. You have a purpose."

I can only ascertain that the state decided to send me to foster care because of what was going on. Abandoned by both parents, neglected, and for unknown reasons, none of my biological fathers' relatives would take me in for the long term. Many possible reasons as to why they did not want to has crossed my mind over the years. Perhaps DFS had questions around why I was given back to my biological donor, who was known to have "problems." While understandably, if a parent requests their child to be given back, the person should comply. However, my thought is if that parent was not of sound mind and known or suspected to be doing drugs, perhaps giving me to that parent would not be safe. Why I did not go back to my Aunt "CeCe" is something I probably will never know. It could be just as simple as she had her own family to take care of and just did not want to deal with another infant. Who knows? DFS possibly felt it was not safe, given that I was handed back to Hildegunde, and that ultimately led to my being left in a house alone and neglected as an infant and deemed not a safe environment. "CeCe" could have also been pissed off at my father for taking off and did not want to be involved in the drama. All plausible. Either way, after the 28 days in ICU, and I was finally medically stable for discharge, and I was placed in foster care. Hildegunde was nowhere to be found. "T" was also MIA. So, I was sent to a nice local family who fostered children. They lived on a farm, and I stayed with them until I was almost two years old. My mom, Andrea, told me that this family loved me. They said that I was happy, sweet, and loved the animals on the farm.

In the interim, my biological father, "T," when travelling with the circus, went to a bar one night with a friend named Giddeon…

18

CHAPTER 2

MOM AND DAD MEET

I was still in foster care in Florida, and the woman I have always regarded as my mom, Andrea, was living in New York at the time. "T" was traveling with the circus and was also in New York at that same time. Previously, I was informed that he and my mom, Andrea, met through a mutual friend and went on a blind date to dinner. However, "T" and Andrea met through Mickey. Andrea and she were friends. Mom says that Mickey told her that she "met these two really cute guys at a bar." Mickey wanted Andrea to be her "wing woman." Mom swears that I was meant to be hers because of all the events that followed. Andrea, who is not one to "party" and definitely would not be found at a bar, agreed to go with Mickey to meet these guys. Mom said they all hung out there and then went back to "continue hanging out" at her place. Mom informed me that from then on, "T" did not return to the circus. Supposedly, he stayed with her. During that time, Mom said that as they were getting to know each other, "T" mentioned that he had a daughter. Since he was gone, he had no idea where I was. Around that time, Steve, "T's" brother, called and asked my biological father, "Where the hell had he been? DFS is looking for you." It was then that Steve informed him that Hildegunde had abandoned me and left me in a house alone, and I had become critically ill as a result, spending nearly a month in the ICU, and was now in foster care. I always wonder how he felt and what he thought at that time when Steven informed him of these things. Guilt? Remorse?

Fear? Or self-serving, narcissistic thoughts blaming everyone else to avoid the spotlight pointing to him?

My mom, Andrea, says to this day, "Nikki, you were meant to be mine because sight unseen, after I heard about you, I wanted you. I had to have you no matter what." She admits that initially, she never wanted children. However, after hearing about me, she wanted me. Mom stated shortly after "T" spoke with Steve, she called Grandma Arlene. Now, if you picture Judge Judy, that was Arlene. They could have been twins! Arlene was a tough cookie, and when Mom called Arlene to tell her about me, Grandma didn't fight it. Mom always says how odd this was. She was expecting Arlene to say, "What are you nuts? You're living with some guy you met at a bar? Get your head out of your ass!" Instead, Grandma agreed. No fight. No resistance. Arlene was living in Florida at the time, while Andrea and "T" were residing in NY. Both Andrea and Arlene worked tirelessly to locate me in the foster system.

"T" and Andrea lived together for about a year. They quickly decided to get married so that Mom could adopt me. For that to happen, they had to put an ad out to inform Hildegunde. Information is limited, but apparently, she popped back in briefly. She was aware that Andrea wanted to adopt me. Just as fast as she came in, she was gone. I have no idea what she knew or said, or anything. I was located on the farm with the foster family and flown to NY, where my biological father and my to-be-adopted mom, Andrea, obtained custody of me. Mom wholeheartedly admits to me that she married "T" for me. "Sight unseen. I can't explain it. I just knew I wanted you," she said. I was flown from FL to NY to meet my parents, and my mom says, "Nikki, I'll never forget it. You got off the plane wearing little overalls with a safety pin holding one of the straps together. You were the cutest thing I've ever seen." I envision Paddington Bear whenever she brings this up. She said that the foster family I was with loved me. They took really good care of me.

My parents ended up relocating, and we drove down to Florida from NY. They resided here for about a year before they married. When I think back, I don't remember the farm at all, and I have a dim memory of the plane trip. But what I do remember was the car ride. It was hot, I was curled in the back seat, and I very specifically remember stopping on the side of the road. I remember a police officer, and in my memory, we were pulled over by him. When I asked about that, my mom said, "No, we just got a flat tire, and the police officer came to help." This is a strong early memory because I remember begging the cop, "Please, don't take my mommy and daddy away." I must have been very traumatized from the initial abandonment, even at that age, to have that response. The only thing I can think of why I responded that way is that I was afraid I was going to lose what I finally desired, my own family. Nothing else about that ride stands out.

"T" and Andrea were married for about eight to nine years and had my sister Samantha when I was six. Eventually, they realized they weren't going to make it as a couple and divorced. Mom says that she wanted to divorce him because she could not take the lies, and he was having a hard time keeping a job. My sister and I went with Mom. The courts appointed custody to her with visitation to him. For a long time, I felt my biological father had gone off to start a new life with his new girlfriend. I guess he wanted to get a second chance at a family other than ours. I do not think that he will ever admit, out loud or even to himself, that we reminded him of his past and a part of him wanted to move forward. Or run away from it. A small piece of me thinks, who can blame him? But you can't run from the past. It will always catch up. You can disillusion others, but not when you face yourself in the mirror.

We were living at Boca Rio when they divorced, and we moved from Boca Rio back to the trailer we had lived in when we were younger. It was purchased not long after Mom and "T" relocated down to FL. In the divorce, Mom kept the trailer, so we had that as a fallback and moved there. It was two bedrooms, and the area in Boca where it was located was nice at that time. Our neighbors became family. Back then, it was that kind of neighborhood where everyone looked out for everyone. The kind of place where you can play outside until the streetlights come on, and also the place I found that paper in the closet that changed everything.

My dad was basically your typical deadbeat dad; all the broken promises, no support, financial or otherwise. I remember sitting on the front porch one afternoon, and my mother's best friend, whom I call Aunt Lorraine, remembers specifically a time when I was so excited to go with Dad for the weekend. She used to always bring this up. "T" was supposed to come and pick me up, and the plan was to go to Lion Country Safari. I must have been around six to seven-years-old. I sat for hours on the steps of the front porch waiting for him, getting excited when a car would go by just to be disappointed when it was not him. Hours went by. He never showed. I remember crying while Lorraine tried to comfort me. He never bothered to call to say anything or explain his absence.

Unfortunately, this became a routine occurrence. Disappointment after disappointment. But I loved him anyway. I excused and believed those excuses. In my eyes, why would he lie? Remember, I did not know about anything at this time. All I knew was that Mommy and Daddy were not together for some reason. Most of my life, I yearned for his approval and love, as all daughters want from their father. While he may have done the best he could, based on what he knew, I do not think he genuinely considered what he was doing inadvertently to my sister and me by being absent, making excuses and how that was destroying our trust for him and its impact for the future relationships we would have, platonic or otherwise. I've contemplated many reasons and even excuses as to why. Perhaps he thought we would be better off? When I was older, I asked him why he did things like that to us. As always, he had some half-assed excuse. It was always somebody else's fault. His job needed him, or he was sick, or some unknown, vague obligation. It was always about him. No apology; no accountability.

Just what he needed to do to get his life together. Yet, for years, I still excused his behavior. After every letdown, I was told by many family members in my life that "T" doesn't take responsibility for his own actions. I know he too was living in "survival mode" but that doesn't mean much to a child who is hurting and feeling abandoned. All she wanted was the love of her father. That's it. To be seen. Looking back, knowing most of the story, I would have thought that given all that happened, and he was given a second chance at being a father, he would have taken that seriously. Instead, his narcissism took center stage. Every time.

As I've gotten older, honestly, I think he developed this self-preserving shield and all of the pathologic lies and excuses were because he would not have been able to look at himself in the mirror, realizing all the things that he had done. So he created stories in his head and to others so that he could face himself every day and not be seen in a bad light. I guess saying that out loud for so long to everyone, you believe your own stories creating an alternate reality where you are the victim. But reality outside his stories was very different...

SUPER STEVEN

Steven was amazing. When my sister and I first met him, we were naturally cautious about him. Remember that at that point, I didn't know the truth of things. Ultimately, there was still hope that my parents were going to get back together, yet we ended up moving into a nice villa in Pompano, Florida, with Steven. My mom met Steven through a mutual friend, who might have been a cousin of Steven's. Ironically, that's how they connected, not unlike how she met my biological father. She and Steven didn't have any children together, and they focused on us girls. Steven never wanted kids of his own. Truth is, Steven told me the same thing Mom did. "Nikki, I never wanted kids. I never did. But that's how I knew that you were meant to be mine, because I wanted you after meeting your mom."

His reasoning for not wanting his own children stemmed from some severe mental disorders and physical ailments within his family. He too suffered from some issues, but not nearly to the degree of his brother, David, who ultimately committed suicide from severe depression. His sister, Laurene, whom I care for, is 59 years old and is in an assisted living facility, suffering from serious medical issues. Because of this, he never wanted to pass those genes on to another. Steven and I got off to a rough start, well, mid mid-start. I gave him hell when I was a teen. Through the years, we became close. He was incredibly humble and loved our family so much. Steven saved us. Steven adopted my sister and me when I was about 12 or so. "T" was not paying child support, and despite mom lowering it and clearing what he had not previously paid because he was always between jobs, he didn't pay. Before meeting Steven, Mom had been doing all she could to care for us. Three jobs and trying to help "T" when he couldn't pay his obligations. Mom took him back to court, and on this last time, according to the paperwork, the judge said to him, "Mr. C, either you pay, or you go to jail." While this seems harsh, remember "T" had barely held up his end of the parental obligations. So, this was not the first offense nor was it the first time having been to court. At the time, Steven had wanted to adopt my sister and me. So, Steven said, "Your honor, if he doesn't want them, I will take them." I have always honored, loved, and respected what he said. Here was a man who never wanted to have his own biological children and took on my mom and her two children to have as his own. I do not think Steven ever realized how special that was to me. Being born into a family that seemingly didn't want me, now here was a man who *chose* me. That is love. That is a father. "T" had an opportunity to step up. What do you think he decided? He did not choose my sister or me. He chose himself. Again.

I remember "T" and I had a conversation about changing my last name. He would tell you that he "only agreed" to my changing my last name to Steven's from "T's" because I agreed to go back to my original last name when I was 18 years old. Sure, perhaps that conversation took place, but do you really think that a daughter who has been searching her whole life thus far for her father's approval would say no? Especially so young. Not only was I looking for his love and acceptance, but I also didn't want to hurt him. Further, in the short time I had known Steven, he had been more of a father than "T". Steven chose us. No rose-colored glasses, and all the baggage didn't matter. He chose us. When opportunities presented themselves to step up, be the rock, the dad we needed, he did. Even though all the shit I gave him. I do believe that subconsciously, I was testing Steven. Perhaps unknowingly trying to push him away because nothing ever stayed. All I knew was disappointment and loss, so I protected my heart. I was afraid to get close. Regardless, Steven stayed. Through all the shit. I do believe at times he even put his own happiness on the back burner so he could be present for us. "T" felt I would have changed my name back at 18. Again, maybe that was how he faced things? I am not sure. But, even if there was a small sense of truth, why would I? What have you done to deserve that? Have you earned it? I had been searching for a sense of family and belonging for as long as I can remember, and "T" repeatedly choosing everything else except my sister and me is not deserving of us to carry his name. So no, I did not.

Now, Steven was a pain in the ass at times. Man was he stubborn! He had such a dry sense of humor and a heart of gold. His laugh was warm and vivacious. He was so intelligent and had a logical and calming approach to things. We did not always see eye to eye, but we respected each other. He stayed through it all. Even when I resisted, he was steadfast, loving, provided a home, and loved us girls so much. It was evident in all he did.

I miss my dad; we lost Steven in 2018. He passed away from complications of multiple myeloma nine days after his 59th birthday. I ultimately diagnosed my stepfather's cancer. The hospital he initially presented himself to, unfortunately, did not see the bigger picture. I professionally advocated for my dad, and I was right. When he was stable, he was discharged from the other hospital, and I brought him to mine. Our hematology and oncology teams were amazing with him. He was responding to treatment. Dad told me that I saved his life. I am not sure about that, but it was the very least I could do after all he had done for me. At the end of 2018, when he passed, my heart broke. I felt such a loss and questioned what I may have "missed" leading to his death. He was doing fantastic. He had just gotten the news that he was a candidate for the bone marrow transplant and was coming off dialysis because his kidney function returned. He became a grandpa as my niece Arlene was born. I will never forget the day he passed. I was working full-time for two departments in the hospital and taking care of him. Further, there was some bullying going on as well, where an anonymous colleague filed a complaint about me. Going through possibly losing my job, while working in two departments and taking care of my dad, really tested me in a lot of ways. I thought I was going to break. My heart is broken, and here everything I worked for was on the line. Thankfully, the work thing worked out, and the investigation revealed that things were not what they were assumed to be. But this would be the last Thanksgiving, the last Hanukkah, and the last birthday I would spend with him. The fragility of life became something I felt. To my core. I would now see November through January very differently moving forward. The fall of 2018 really tested me. It nearly broke me. Steven's passing left a void in my heart. Different from when Grandpa Larry passed, but just as empty. What I did not want to do this time was push everyone away the way I did when Grandpa passed. What I am thankful for is that Dad passed on his terms. He was home, received great news that day about the above, and had a grandchild. In the Jewish religion, it is believed that the closer a person passes to the end of the year, the more fulfilled their life was. That gave me some comfort because Steven deserved to be at peace.

As I look back and I see where I'm at now, honestly, up until recently, I never really understood what the impact of all that was and how fortunate I am to have those around me that I genuinely feel were strategically placed every step of the way. My entire life, the universe has purposefully placed people in my life that would trigger me one way or the other, and also to support and help me.

I am reminded of this each time I look in the mirror and see the residual scar from the central line when I was a *failure to thrive* when I was in the hospital. And like it or not, I carry the trauma from those scars with me. Although I was too young to remember consciously, they are always there under the surface. Each piece of the puzzle I've uncovered about my story has laid, or shall I say, strengthened the foundation of who I am. Mom says, "God made a mistake," but I have to question that. Did he really? Or was this the plan the whole time?

CHAPTER 3

LETTING THE NEGATIVE OUTWEIGH THE POSITIVE

Much of my life I wanted to know why I wasn't lovable. I couldn't allow myself to wrap my head around the fact that no matter how my life began, the outcome was actually positive. I took my family dynamics as negative, and in fact, I saw that as negative for most of my life. When I was told about Hildegunde abandoning me and that she was my biological mother, I felt betrayed. I was so sad with all of that was going on, I shaved off my eyebrows and pulled out all my eyelashes. I didn't want anybody to see the expression on my face. The sadness and anxiety I suffered with for a long time. For much of my life, I did not really tell anyone how I felt. I reasoned that I was already "damaged," and if people really knew my story or how I was feeling, that would further isolate me. The reality is that thought is self-destructing. One that many feel. Often, we bury it because we don't want to "bother" anyone or be seen in a poor light.

I was really angry and looking to lash out at every turn. For a long time. I had trust issues and didn't make friends easily. Believe it or not, I am very much an introvert. During that time, I was sullen and distant all through middle school, but when we moved to Boca from Blue Lake, I saw that as a fresh start and wanted to try to make friends. For no apparent reason, one of the girls on the block started bullying me. I guess because I was the new kid and she felt threatened in some way? Who knows? Kids can be so cruel to one another. This was just one of many bullies I would encounter throughout my life. Her behavior added to my trust issues. I kept most everybody at arm's length. I will test you. Not on purpose. But, to see if you stay. Arm's length feels safer. I don't like feeling vulnerable. I tend to do that even to this day, though I've gotten a lot better with it. I was really reluctant to let people in growing up, so, instead, I would just act out. I ran the usual gamut of troubled teen angst, skipping school, sneaking out, experimenting with drugs, drinking, boys, all the stuff, but what I think kind of tipped it over the edge was the bullying. These events contributed to my distancing myself, smoking pot, etc. It was almost as if I saw it as confirmation of how I felt unlovable, damaged.

It was spring or early summer when we moved into the new neighborhood, and soon middle school started. During Christmas break, Christine, one of the girls who liked to bully me, had a party. I got invited with the other kids on the block, and after the party, she accused me of stealing her watch. I was still a relatively new student at this school and was slowly beginning to make a few friends, but now I was labeled as a thief. I was embarrassed. I wanted to move. She spread all kinds of rumors around about me and made me out to be a terrible person. Here I had an opportunity to "begin again," yet other plans were in place. As it turned out, her mom had just taken the watch to the jeweler to get it sized and cleaned. Despite that, Christine just kept on talking me down at every turn. I do remember an apology, but to others, at school, she stood firm in the bullying behavior. In fact, even encouraged it. I am not really sure what I ever did to her.

I remember an event when I was into smoking pot at that point and often smoked with a boy named Jimmy. A good friend of mine, or so I thought, Diana, had a crush on Jimmy. Christine and Diana were talking and decided to tell Jimmy's girlfriend that he and I hung out smoking. Maybe Diana thought that it would break them up, and she could swoop in and have a chance with him? Christine lied to Jimmy's girlfriend and said that I was not just hanging out smoking, but that I was hooking up with him. I was still a virgin at that time, and I wasn't into doing any of that. We were just smoking pot. That was all we had in common. I was playing hockey at school and was your typical tomboy. Climbed trees, played sports, I was not acting slutty. I took to shaving the back of my head and sneaking out my bedroom window at night, but I wasn't having sex and certainly not with Jimmy. But thanks to Christine's lies, when I was walking home from school one afternoon, three guys and a girl jumped me, I guess to "teach me" a lesson about stealing someone's boyfriend.

I remember just lying on the ground and being kicked and punched. They tried to take a ring off my finger that my grandma Arlene gave me. It was an heirloom. And I always say, thank God I cracked my knuckles because it didn't come off right away. The guy I was dating, John, and I would usually meet up on my way home at the bus loop where he would pick me up. My luck, that day he happened to be running behind and was a few minutes late picking me up. But one of my good friends at the time, James, who I played street hockey with, happened to be passing by on his bike. James and I would compete against the other neighborhoods, and one time, he rolled over onto one of the drainage grates and broke both of his wrists, so he had short arm casts on both broken wrists.

Luckily, he was riding his bike home at that exact moment and saw me getting kicked and punched by all these people. James hopped off his bike and jumped into the fight. He stopped me from getting seriously injured. This kid, who had two broken wrists, was somehow able to pick up his bike and throw it at these people. It was beyond belief. I uncovered my head, slowly peeked up and right after he did that, a blue car rolled up. I think they were friends with James, but I am not sure. I got in the car with them, and then, we saw John. I got out of that car, got into John's and ultimately, we went to the police station in Mission Bay, where I filed a report. The people in the blue car went to find those people. I remember looking across the street just before it happened and saw Diana. I thought it was odd she didn't say hello. She just watched.

When all that happened, something snapped in my brain and a part of me thought, *you know what? Why don't I just fit the mold? If this is what all these people think of me, then why don't I just become that?* I wanted to give up. I felt defeated. Hopeless.

I was lost for a long time. My adolescent and teenage years were not happy times for me, none of it. I got jumped a second time, some months later, with Christine and Jimmy's girlfriend showing up at my house just after trying to pick a fight with me on the way home from school. Home life was not good; Mom and Steven were fighting. My sister would try to get me into trouble for things I never even did. I ended up dropping out of high school and moving out of my home. I left home and had roommates the first time when I was 16, almost 17, and I dropped out the first time my sophomore year, and my mom said, "Well, if you're not going to school, you're going to work because you're going to pay rent." I don't remember what the rent she wanted to charge me was, but she came up with a ridiculous number that I could not in a million years be able to pay. I tried for a little while, but that didn't work. So, thinking I was smart and could live elsewhere on my own, I moved out. Epic fail, and ultimately, I came back just before I turned 17.

I didn't last long trying to go back to high school and eventually dropped out again as a junior. I was going to do night school, but after being jumped, I did not feel safe going to school no matter what I tried. So I would skip a lot. I was skipping before, but now it was every day rather than a class or two. My mom would drop me off, and then I would just walk right out the bus loop. I don't think she had any idea.

So, I was nearly 17, a dropout, and not sure what I was going to do with my life. My mom pressured me to get my GED. It was not something I wanted to do, but she made it clear that it was not an option. She wanted me to become something and knew I could. My biological father, on the other hand, would always tell me that I was going to be barefoot and pregnant. Those were the actual words that he would use. Thanks, Dad, but Mom would say, "No, you're not. You are going to have a much better future." So, I tried night school, but I just felt like the walls were closing in. I couldn't go. And I lied to my mom about it. I told her I was going, and I wasn't. Finally came clean and told her. Then, I signed up for the GED at Boca High, took it, and passed. At that point, I was almost 18. Shortly after that, I moved out of the house again. My mom and I did not get along at that point because she was not in a good place at that time either. She was doing school full-time, and Steven was working. She wasn't happy with who she was. And I have to say, though, even with all of that, the running joke in the family is that I raised her. Our situation at that time was toxic. We both said things to each other that were awful. She was miserable, and I was too. I felt like an outcast in my own life. No self-love, not sure I even saw a future. The darkness was real. I began believing what these other people thought, and the darkness tried to creep in permanently.

I am so incredibly proud of her even though we didn't get along for a bit, because I was stuck in my life, and had a really hard time seeing the positive. I was carrying around all these burdens. I just figured nobody loved me, even though my mom absolutely did. That's the crazy part. The truth is that I went from having no family to a family that chose to take me and put up with my shit my whole life. There's got to be something really special in that. They didn't have to take me, especially as "damaged" as I was. Then though, I couldn't see the good in all that, only the betrayal and abandonment.

While I was rebelling and making things hard for myself and my family, Mom was growing and doing her own stuff. We were both just miserable, and that was ultimately why I ended up leaving.

My sister was getting older too, and was being a little asshole and trying to get me in trouble for everything. So what was the reason to stay? I do remember entertaining the feeling that Mom favored Sam because they were "blood." Even though that was why Sam was such a jerk to me. I did not see that I belonged. The weight of everyone's burdens blinded me.

I was just lost and miserable, and I felt like I had nothing, and I just couldn't see any sort of light. All I could think was, *you know what? I just gotta get out of here*. When I left that time, at almost 18, I stayed out. I stayed with friends, couch surfed, and hopped around a little bit for a time. I stayed with a guy who was a good friend of mine at that time, Frankie. And other people here and there, but Frankie was the one I stayed with the longest.

Over the years, I had various roommates here and there. I would tag along with them, but that's ultimately what it was. As for work, I did a little bit of everything. I worked for Albertsons as a cashier. I did some work at a pottery store. I also dressed up as characters like Bart Simpson, a ninja turtle, and Barney at local craft fairs. That was one of my first jobs, Blockbuster too. I tried my hand at waitressing, doing whatever I could to make money. Never anything illegal, though. I didn't do anything like that. I sold shots at a bar and at the strip club, wherever I could make money. One of the guys I met through a mutual friend at the bar I was working at I ended up dating, was named Jeremy. He was trash. Oddly enough, his sister had the same first name and middle name as me, but with a different last name. This little fact is pertinent because they went on a spending spree using my credit information. That was fun!

I was 19 or 20 and had done a couple of years of bouncing around when I had what I would call my wake-up moment. I was dating all the wrong guys. I was looking for love in all the places where love does not exist. I was dating a guy named John at the time, and my friend Michelle was dating John's brother, Anthony. Another roomie I had, we will call him "Fred," told me earlier in the day, that he had feelings for me. I didn't have those same feelings, and he got upset. Now we had been roommates for a while. Perhaps he thought things were different? When I didn't reciprocate his feelings, he put his hands on my neck, and I blew a circuit. He and I had some very choice words, and I called "Michi," crying about the unexpected incident. Looking in the mirror, tears running down my face with finger marks on my neck, I asked her if I could come over to her place. I needed to decide what to do because now, my living arrangements no longer felt safe.

"If you're going to come over and stay here, you've got a party with us," was her response. I needed to get out of there and that's ultimately what happened. We were drinking and smoking pot. I vaguely remember taking some sort of pills. One minute, I was standing in the middle of the living room, and the next thing I knew, I woke up on the floor with blood dripping down the side of my face. I didn't know where the blood had come from. Maybe I had overdosed? This might sound crazy, but I managed to get to my feet, leave Michi's, and drive myself to the nearest hospital. I was so scared. When I was admitted, I told the doctor, "I drank, I smoked, and I took some pills. I woke up with blood on my face, and I don't know if it came from my mouth, my ear, my nose, I have no idea." They did the whole charcoal thing. They took labs and after all the tests, they said everything was fine.

And that moment for me was what I call my *apple moment*. Because I thought about that saying *the apple doesn't fall far from the tree. Well, oh no, this apple is going way across the Pacific, as far away from the tree that was my bio-mom.* I felt like it was a flash of her. Knowing all I did about her, seeing my life at this moment, I was *not* repeating history. I was better than that. Than all of this. The light was beginning to creep in. The embers were lit.

Pain to Power

CHAPTER 4

EMBERS BEGIN TO MULTIPLY

The universe definitely placed people in my life and showed me signs that everything ultimately would be okay. There were a lot of uphill battles, a lot of catalysts for me to go down really dark roads, and there were also a lot to counter that as well. Growing up through all of this, I did go down some pretty dark paths, but I could have easily gone and stayed there. I would always be brought to the thought that I didn't want to be like her. I didn't want to be like him. I didn't want to make the same mistakes. I was breaking this mold. This apple was going way across the ocean. Randomly, and I am not even sure where these fleeting embers of light would creep into my thoughts, but each time they showed themselves, it brought me one step closer to the flame.

I have encountered bullying every step of the way. There have been *many,* even to this day, who have tried to put my fire out. It seemed there was always some catalyst trying to push me down the dark roads. Looking back, it is almost as if there were test after test; the universe putting these obstacles in my way to see how I would handle them. Or perhaps this was a preparation for something? Many times I nearly caved and contemplated how life would be if I were not around. Even if I temporarily succumbed to the dark side, where even the sense of direction was unable to be seen, I would not stay. *I couldn't.* These embers would light the way.

I remember working for one Diagnostic Center where I had my first recognition that mean girl groups exist even in the professional atmosphere. After I graduated with my ultrasound degree, I thought that I was just going to be able to get started with life. Ha, joke was on me. All I wanted was to be able to move forward and get on a good path. But the universe had other plans...

I scheduled the time to take the boards for ultrasound, which are incredibly difficult. One of them is all physics, acoustical physics. The other is whatever specialty you choose. I chose to take the abdominal board, which has pediatrics in it and covers all the abdominal organs, like a general medicine kind of a board for ultrasound. That's usually the most common one to take.

I scheduled both of those two on the same day, not knowing what the heck I was getting myself into. I can truthfully say that I underestimated them. Definitely bit off more than I could chew. I thought I studied enough, and I just wanted to just move forward and get life started, begin my new path. In my mind, I had gone through so much already, and I was ready to get going on all things positive. Not realizing that perhaps *my timing* was not right. As you can imagine, I was very insecure about all things academic, given dropping out of school, so perhaps I was blinded by the gravity of the situation. I took the boards and failed them both. Miserably. I completely underestimated the situation. I remember after sitting for the physics board first and after question 15, my neurons were shot. I was brain-dead and filled with anxiety. Well, the complete emotional response and loss of control are why I failed. I got intimidated. Felt like an imposter.

After I left the testing center, I was like, *What the hell did I do to myself?* I was so embarrassed, and I thought that people were going to look down on me so, **I lied about it**. I told people that I had passed, but the paper blew out the window. I came up with this kind of shit not to feel ashamed of myself. Even though secretly, I was beating myself up inside. After graduation, I got hired at a local hospital for ultrasound. I was approaching my year there and in order to maintain your job you had to pass your ARDMS boards (two of them) within that year as a new graduate. It was my first job out of school. So, even though I had failed, I was still within that year time frame. I thought, *okay, I'll just take it again and then nobody will know I failed the first time.*

I took the boards a second time and failed them a second time. This really stung. I thought I did things right and studied. Well, the test anxiety crept in and so did my insecurity for all things academic. Imposter syndrome took center stage and coupled with my anxiety is why I failed. But I refused to give up. I would pass and become certified.

On my third attempt, I finally got it right, but by then I had to leave the job because I didn't make the one-year deadline. I had already anticipated this, and I was looking for another job. From there, I went to another hospital in Aventura. I didn't mind leaving the first hospital because there was too much toxicity in the department, especially among the "mean girl clan." Even some of the managers there were nasty and just plain mean humans. Here, this was my second "big girl" job, and I was not impressed. I remember thinking to myself, *why do I keep encountering these types of people? Why can't I just find friends who have the same goals? To live a life we love. No drama. No excuses. Supporting each other.* I couldn't put my finger on it. I could not figure out why I kept encountering these situations. Perhaps it was the universe's way of teaching me? I already felt alone and like no one understood, and yet still encountered toxicity. I felt like I just couldn't win.

TRUE LOVE VS. SELF LOVE

At the first hospital, I met one of the sonographers, named "D". We began dating, and I loved him. It was a different feeling from John. I respected the man he was, even the parts he tried to hide.

He is a fantastic sonographer. He was the first man that I thought we were going to be together forever, but unfortunately it didn't work out that way. He is a good man. He has a good heart, but it is closed off. Unknowingly, he was the first man to show me what I did not want. He always held me at arm's length, and despite dating for a few years, that never changed. Despite everything I had been through with love, one would think that I would be toxic and needy. But if anything, it was the opposite. I will give you enough rope to hang yourself, and I did that with him. Possibly too much so. I was a people pleaser at that time, so I fully am aware that my distance may have confused things and made it feel like it was okay to keep me at a distance. Because I, too, was afraid to be vulnerable. Or perhaps it was almost as if I was expecting to be let down because that was all I knew. What I do know is that I had let my guard down with him, so much so that I even said "I love you." He was the first person I had said that to. I can recall the exact moment everything changed with him.

Now remember, I, too, am very guarded, so at first, it was just a "friends with benefits" situation that evolved into more. Maybe he held on to me and vice versa because it was simple? Drama-free? Not sure, but I know he also had trust issues. After a couple of years of dating, there was a hurricane that was supposed to hit. He and I were trapped in the house for a few days together. Slowest hurricane ever! I was thinking, *maybe this is the time to tell him how I feel?* Before then, I had not told him. I was really feeling the "itch" to tell him.

At first, I chickened out. Vulnerability sucks, and so does rejection. Finally, after two days of being in the house, the coast was clear, and the storm passed. A bunch of us went out to celebrate, had some food and drinks. One of "D's" friends, Marco, and I had chatted about "D" and my feelings for him. Marco encouraged me to tell him how I felt. I respected Marco. From his perspective, "D" would react positively to it. I decided to go for it after some convincing that it was safe to open up. *Okay, here goes I thought.*

We all left the restaurant, arriving at "D's", and as we were walking to the front door, I said it. "I love you." His reaction was not at all what I was expecting. He got annoyed and notably upset. I don't remember his initial words, but I remember that I was hurt. I began tearing up in front of Marco and his other friend, Tony. "D" looked at me and said, "I don't love you, and I don't need this drama." *Wait. What?! Oh, no. The first time I let my guard down to a man and express how I feel, and this is what happens? Saying it so loudly that both Tony and Marco heard it.*

I was mortified. I punched the wall. It was brick. I remember having acute pain in my wrist, but the adrenaline that was flowing quieted it. I collected my things after an argument and went back to my apartment. Well, "D's" apartment. I had moved into his old apartment because he was having a hard time renting it. It was convenient for both at that time. Rent was fair, and my other lease was up. We kept it professional. No mixing of the emotions. Just business surrounding the apartment. Official documents drawn and all. I didn't want any confusion or boundary crossing on either end. This situation was the turning point for me. Even if he didn't mean it, saying what he said would never allow him the keys to my heart again. I couldn't feel safe with him. Ever.

One might say, "Maybe he didn't know about your past," or find some other way to defend his words, but no. He knew. I could never trust him again. Ultimately, that was the end of the relationship. When the lease ended, I moved out and eventually back to Broward County. He did try to make up for his words, but with all that I have already been through, I could not trust my heart with him. I did try briefly. But I never saw him the same again. That situation reinforced the wall that had already been up. I am, even to this day, someone who if you cross that boundary and betray me, there is no going back. I don't mean small things. People can differ in opinions, and disagreement is healthy. But, if I can't trust you or your loyalty to our friendship/relationship is questioned, I don't come back. I choose me. I don't do drama exits either. I just walk away, protecting my peace. This was definitely something he could not come back from. I realized I would have always had questions and then would have resented him. He does not deserve that kind of "love," and neither do I. So, I let him go.

I chose self-love as my true love...

CHAPTER 5

A DIFFICULT DECISION

Before "D" and I started dating, I had dated this guy, Lynn. He had two daughters of his own from his first marriage. We met when I was waiting tables at TGI Friday's. Lynn and I were dating before I graduated from ultrasound school. We dated for a few years. I liked him. There was always this issue of age though. Lynn was about eight years older than I was. I wasn't bothered by it, but he was. Especially because one of his "friends" and his family would routinely bring this up to him. Honestly, I think his friend Ashley did this because she was in love with him, and she continued to try to drive a wedge between us. Lynn didn't know that I knew. Plus, they had been together previously. But he was with me now, or so I thought.

Quite honestly, I always felt they still had something going on, but I would dismiss it because I thought I was being paranoid. Eventually, Lynn suggested that we move in together. At that time, I was renting a room from Katie in Hollywood. She was a great roommate. The lease was ending, and though I was reluctant to move in with Lynn, I did it. He was very convincing, and it appeared that he wanted long term. He didn't want me to live on my own and have to pay rent while in school. So, he just said, "Come live with me." Well, little did I know that my mom was giving him money every month from my student loans to help with my expenses. I don't know how that arrangement happened. I don't know if my mom offered it. I don't know if he asked for it. I have no idea, but she was giving him some of the student loan money. This fact is important for a lot of reasons, but the main reason was that was my first awakening to the fact that not everybody and not everything is what it may seem.

I got pregnant from Lynn just around the time I graduated from ultrasound program. I had so many mixed feelings. *How do I tell him? I already hate being vulnerable, and now I will be permanently be tied to him. Would he be happy about it? Would I be?* The insecure and perhaps intuitive feelings about Lynn and Ashley still remained. So, I was not really sure how he would react. To me, we had a happyish life together. But was that enough? I was helping to take care of his kids, who I adored. The girls are amazing. Erika was cautious of me, and I could understand why. I was not her mom, nor was I trying to replace her. Eventually, she and I bonded. I stood by Lynn's side through everything. I do not want to put his business out there, but let's just say, a very bad situation occurred through no fault of his own. Regardless, I stayed by him, supporting how I could.

With all the ups and downs, I figured he might be happy about the pregnancy. Plus, I was just about to graduate from ultrasound school so there would be extra income. I thought that there should not be anything he wouldn't be happy about unless my intuition was correct, and he was having an affair with Ashley. I mustered up the strength to tell him. I will never forget the face he made. It was one of fear and disappointment. Not one of joy. He was so annoyed that I had gotten pregnant, as if it were my fault alone. We lived together and he had every opportunity to discuss his feelings, but for over a week, he said nothing about it. Avoided me and it. Talk about a knife to the heart. He wouldn't discuss it. He kept pushing it off. All sorts of thoughts and emotions were going through my head. *Here we are again. Another disappointment. What do these men want from me? A good time, apparently, but without the commitment.*

Shortly after, I remember a specific event that promoted and provoked conversation, illuminating the reality of the situation. One day, we went to the grocery store, and it got weird. Really weird. I asked Lynn, "Hey, can you grab me some Cheerios?" He just kind of looked at me and said, "No, I'll grab you what I want." It was just the way that it had come out of his mouth, and I was thinking to myself, *I never want to be in a position where I'm financially responsible to someone or have somebody be financially responsible for me.*

When we got home, this revealed the whole reality. Mom was giving Lynn money, AND he WAS having an affair. But not with Ashley. *Whoa, what? The heck?! And here I was, pregnant with his child?! No way. I am not staying in this situation.* I was devastated. Here was a man who said he "loved" me and who prompted and led the whole relationship, who was sleeping around and had some secret business deal with my mom! No, thank you. Talk about betrayal. I was enraged. I had never felt anything like that. I grabbed the scissors and went to the bathroom. I made so many cuts on my arms and thighs. I just wanted the pain to stop. *Why can't anyone love me? Why? Why do I keep being discarded?* Lynn refused to talk about the pregnancy. So, I made the decision.

He refused to talk to me about it for about a week. I did one of the cruelest things that I could do. The way that I thought about it was, *if you can't be a man to talk to me about it, I'm making the decision myself. You're sleeping with another woman and keeping secrets?* I chose to have an elective abortion. He was pro-life, so I knew that was going to affect him, and I didn't care. *You can't talk to me? You can knock me up, but you can't talk to me for over a week, and we live in the same house?* I realized he was not the kind of person I wanted around me or to raise a child with. I live with that decision every day. But, I was not going to be a statistic. I did not want a child to be caught in the middle of this. I did not want to bring a child into this world who could potentially be made to feel like an outcast, to feel rejected or abandoned. What would I have told him or her growing up? I know exactly what it feels like, and it is an awful weight on your heart. I could not choose to do that to another.

Very shortly after that, I moved out. I had the procedure, recovered, and then left. This almost sent me down a dark spiral, but it turned out that the reason he was so conflicted was that he had been cheating on me with another woman nearly the whole time we were together. That was why he couldn't talk to me about it. Because he would have had to reveal all these details. To both of us. He was selfish. Not for one second was he thinking of how I was feeling. All that mattered was how it would look and how he could explain it. To her, me, and his family. He tried to make things right with me after I moved out. I was very attached to his daughters, and that hurt. His girls were amazing. He was close with my grandma, Arlene, and he called her often. I don't feel that the attempts, even to this day, were genuine. It was just to clear his conscience.

One day, several months later, he called me, and I don't know if it was revenge, but he called to inform me that he was getting married and *invited me to their wedding*. He was marrying the girl he cheated on me with. I lost my shit. I don't even know what I said, but I was so angry, and I was thinking to myself, *Are you kidding me? Like, seriously, this is what you're doing?* I was irate. I felt destroyed. I did feel unstable. He must have felt it too because never had I behaved that way before.

Under the guise of concern, he called my grandma and told her that he was worried that I was going to take my own life. I might be a lot of things. I might get sad, angry, disappointed, and may not have had the most self-love at that time, but he was not that special no matter what he thought of himself. I would never give all my power away to him. Everything I had already been through and survived, and this would be the tipping point? What he did was cruel. Probably revenge for the abortion. He called Grandma because HE felt bad for potentially provoking a fatal outcome.

That's what it was. It had nothing to do with me. Regardless of his reasons, I would NEVER end my life because of HIS choices. I am stronger than that. Shortly after this, I met "D" Little did I know…

As I learned, "D" didn't want a serious relationship. What erupted from that situation, I feel, was a combination of many different disappointments. Three years with Lynn and then Dennis? I was getting used to being let down and never considered. Not even by myself. I can't blame them for all of it. Yes, what these two did was cruel. They too, were broken. However, I saw the signs, I just refused to acknowledge them. I chose mistreatment. I wanted to be loved so badly that I did not want to see the red flags. I wanted a home. To feel loved, safe, needed, and appreciated. I was looking for love in all the wrong places. Looking back, I didn't even love myself, so how was anyone else going to be able to? I kept accepting less because some part of me felt I deserved it. Carrying the weight of the burdens placed on me by others. I couldn't "see" two feet in front of my face.

Disappointment, job losses, being my own worst enemy, bullying… What is next? I admit I had a role to play in how others treated me. I had a hard time with people in general. I do take responsibility for some of it. I was guarded and standoffish, not because that was what I wanted, but because it was all I knew at that time. It was protection. Survival mode. Everyone I loved, left. I was getting tired of people taking from me, my love, my energy, my time… and leaving. How do you trust anything?

Little did I know that one of the biggest heartbreaks and betrayals was about to occur.

CHAPTER 6

LOSING TRUST IN A DEAR FRIEND

Lisa and I were best friends for over 25 years, but that changed, unfortunately, when I went to PA school. Unless you're in medicine, I don't think people genuinely understand what that entails. The amount of time and dedication, plus the sacrifices made. Anyone in medicine knows we lose time with friends and family for a host of different reasons. Competition to get into the programs is real. It is incredibly difficult. Emotionally taxing. Thousands of applications, and you want them to "see" you on paper. You need to be in the top 10% to gain an interview.

When I was working on getting my bachelor's degree at Barry, I HAD to focus. I had to make up for past educational mistakes. I needed to prove to myself I could. It wasn't enough that I passed my boards for ultrasound and even obtained multiple subspecialties. I needed to prove to myself I was capable. I was scared out of my mind, but I had to do it. Consider this my first real form of self-love.

Shortly after beginning at Barry University, I moved up to Wellington. I was driving from Wellington to Miami five to six times a week to go to school. I had to be very militant and regimented about my schedule. There was an enormous amount of information and coursework that needed to be done. So, I needed to be efficient with my time. Especially driving so far. I had to miss traffic in three counties to make it to classes on time. It was an hour each way without traffic. I woke up each morning at 4:30 a.m., out the door by 6:00 a.m. for classes at 8:00 a.m. There was no room for error or extra things. I just didn't have the time to be physically present for my friends or often even my family. But I was present in other ways. I would call, send things for birthdays, and condolences when appropriate. Some understood and some did not. I had to get in. I had years of GPA mess-ups that I needed to account for. PA programs are incredibly competitive. The average GPA accepted for science and overall GPA is 3.0. But the average GPA to gain an interview at that time was a 3.5 in science and overall. My degree for ultrasound? I was lucky to graduate with barely a 2.8. That meant I needed to get a 4.0 in Barry for the bachelor's to even get close to acceptance, let alone an interview. My GRE, dropping out of school, the bullying and failures at Keiser had all affected my GPA. I needed to prove on paper that I was not a failure. That I was "worthy" of acceptance.

Each semester I took on more. Why? Well, If I was going to put myself through the rigors of PA school, I needed to see if I could handle the pressure. If I couldn't, then why even bother? I began with eight credits, earned a 4.0. Moved to twelve, then sixteen, then finally to twenty-one credits. As I took on more, I also needed to log volunteering and patient care hours to be competitive. So, I tutored biology and chemistry courses, did research, and became a part of some of the clubs. In the beginning, I was also working as an ultrasound tech. My classes were scheduled around my work schedule. I had no time.

For those who have never been through this, all of these things are mandatory for the applications. It was not a "just because." More often than not, I couldn't be physically present in the rest of my life. This rigorous schedule continued for about five years. The first time I applied to PA school, I was not accepted. I was not competitive enough, and I submitted late. This was a complete blow. I remember crying to one of my favorite humans ever, Dr. Bingham.

She was one of my Barry undergraduate professors and research professor who knew all my struggles and who helped me along the way, offering guidance, confidence, and fostering growth within. She is one of the people who I truly believe the universe placed in my path to help me.

When I graduated from Barry University, I graduated summa cum laude, and she was there every step of the way. The year following, after being rejected, I applied again. This time, learning from my mistakes and applying early. After all my prior and recent course-work over a span of ten years, my overall GPA was just barely a 3.4 after being entered into the platform used to apply for PA school. I was so nervous, but finally the interviews came, and so did graduation from Barry University PA Program. Never had I felt more accomplished and so proud of myself. When graduation came, I wanted to have a little celebration with those I loved at a local restaurant. I sent a text to my then-best friend, who I have known since we were five years old, and she did something that cut me to the core. I considered her my sister. We went through so much together. Little did I know....

I sent a group chat out and invited all of the people I was close to in my life to come to my graduation party. I was dating my husband-to-be, Andrew, at the time, and there was a group chat that all the girls in the friend group were in. I texted, *"I know it has been a little while since we hung out. But If you want to come, I'm going to have a little get-together at Rocco's, and I would love to see you all."*

Nothing was wrong that I knew of, but in the chat, Lisa (my now ex-best friend) decided to type *"How desperate!"* to the group chat. I was floored. That message took my breath away and broke my heart. I could not believe what I was reading. I felt my mind was playing tricks on me. I read it over and over hoping it was some hallucination. She definitely messaged that to the wrong group. There was another group chat that I'm sure the other girls were in with her, but I was not. I believe that one of the other girls side-messaged her to inform her about her saying those things in the wrong chat. This was somebody that I thought was with me, my whole life, through thick and thin, my ride or die through all the things. I assumed that this human would tell me if something was wrong, not disrespect me or our friendship. I do think it was a mistake, and when she realized it, she wanted to make it right, to have a discussion.

I heard her out, ultimately, but I didn't understand why she felt reaching out to people who I thought were good friends to celebrate with me was a desperate move. Her excuse was that she felt I wasn't making enough time to be there for her or any of my friends. I reminded her that while more often than not, I could not always physically be there. I tried to make myself present in other ways. I tried to explain my situation to her. I apologized for my role in hurting her because I am sure she felt hurt, and her feelings were valid. But up to that point, she had never said a word, and instead I found out with a weird, random, mistakenly sent to the wrong group "desperate" text! She wasn't one to talk about emotions often, but she did with me. I could not wrap my head around why she never reached out.

I now felt that she was untrustworthy. She felt comfortable sending that message even if it was to the wrong chat, which means she and the other girls were talking shit about me behind my back. Never mentioning how they felt to *me*, I informed her that I barely even saw Andrew and we lived together. We'd been like roommates passing each other in the night for quite some time. "If you felt a certain way, you should have said something to me," I told her. "This should not have been how I find out?" Especially because it was her. I trust very few people in this world, and she was one. She knew all of me, and I thought I did of her. I guess I was wrong.

I was not having it. My mom was furious and shocked that Lisa would behave that way. After that whole sad disappointment, I just didn't want to know her anymore. We had lunch like a year later, but I still could not trust her. I was really hoping that I would feel different. I loved her. She was a piece of my heart. I have forgiven her and assumed responsibility for my part in things, but I don't want someone in my life who behaves that way. After 25 years of sistership, I walked away from her, cut her off, and I have not spoken to her since, and I refuse to do so. She was the *last* person I thought would betray me. I love her, miss her, and want the best for her and her family, but I'll never be able to trust her fully again.

I admit that I hate that I've gotten comfortable with walking away from people and watching others walk away. I don't know if it's a protective mechanism or if it's a realization that, *you know what, that chapter with this individual has run its course. I am grateful for them, thankful for the lesson…*

"On to the next chapter. With the turn of each page, we are built from the love, laughter, and tears of the pages before. With the turn of each page, we are anew. Utilizing lessons learned, we are humbled. We are stronger and built from the flames. We are loved. We are freed. Without resentment or guilt. Without fear. Carrying our journey proudly. Without regrets. With the turn of each page, I willfully soar into the future. Gracefully accepting each challenge and experience that brings me to new heights. Conquering all that is set before me. On to the next chapter, my wings are ready, as you are with me"

Nicole Schtupak, 2019, In memory of Steven, Grandpa Larry, and Grandma Arlene

Power

CHAPTER 7

PUSHING LIMITS

STAYING TRUE TO YOUR CONVICTIONS

As a medical professional, you don't have time to waste on small issues. My students say I am funny because I'm laid back and sarcastic. Sometimes I will shoot off these little quick-witted comments, but when shit gets real, I flip the switch and get down to business. I tell them that is the Gemini in me.

For the last five or six years, the universe has been pushing boundaries on me, and it has been throwing me into the fire in every which way possible to get me to say no and to stop being a people pleaser. It must be working, because recently I cut off my biological father, and I'm starting to see people for who they are instead of what their potential could be. Previously, I would try to find the good in people, and I will still do that, but once you show me who you really are, that's what I need to accept as truth, not who you might become.

For a long time, I had no boundaries, especially with my biological father. His acceptance was what I wanted most, but he lacks insight, accountability, and is a narcissist. Even if he does have some shred of those traits, he buries it, blames everything else, and takes no accountability. He's always the smartest person in the room, and the victim.

I'm very, very, very big on women's rights. I don't know if past lives are genuinely a thing, but if they are, I was definitely the one who was stoned in the square or burned on the stake. I will always stand up for what's right. Especially when it comes to giving a voice to women. I got into medicine, in general, to give a voice to women and to be that voice. It's deeply rooted in me, in my DNA.

I would post vetted things on social media merely just to post it for education and information. I don't want to convince anybody of anything. I want people to just think for themselves. I really don't want my ideas to influence their decisions, just... *here's information. Do what you want with it.* The women's health thing is a big issue especially now with what is happening in this country, and worldwide for that matter. This is serious.

I forget exactly what I posted, but I posted something about women's health, and my biological father, "T" responded in true form with a laughing emoji. When it showed on my feed, I just looked at that damn emoji and thought, *you piece of trash. You have two daughters and a granddaughter, and that's what you're posting? Even if that's really what you think, you physically put that out there to note that you think women's desperate needs for healthcare is a joke.*

That was my tipping point with him. Of all the things, I could not believe it. What is kind of ironic though is that "T" is such a conservative and doesn't believe there should be government assistance for those in need. Well, the government helped support his children when mom was working three jobs, and he was off doing whatever he was, except paying child support. The government did HIS job and took care of his oldest daughter while she was in foster care, and he took off to join the circus because he couldn't face his reality. *So, really, "T"?* Perhaps you should look in the mirror and take accountability before you start placing laughing emojis on your daughter's post.

Well, that is who my father really is. There are no rose-colored glasses to wear to make him someone else. Except he wears them, avoiding the truth and accountability. So, yes, I blocked him everywhere I could. He has had over 40 years to make things right. To prove he genuinely wants to rebuild. Although, those in his life would think I am the enemy. How terrible I am because he has tried to be present. Well, I'm here to say again, no he has not. He has done none of the sort except for half-assed attempts that, in his own mind, are appropriate for concocting a storyline that makes him the victim. He has done less than minimal effort yet wants all of the credit to feed his ego. No. Nor I or my sister owe him anything. The goodness of our hearts has given him ample opportunities, and also probably because of some toxic attachment issues, to be a dad. He has chosen himself each time.

So, out of love for myself, my sister, and my niece, that was my stand. He is removed. Permanently. No drama. No reason. Just done. Now, some may feel a certain way about me not having a conversation with him. Well, my answer to that is if you had ever spoken with him, you'd see he gaslights and manipulates things to take focus off him. I don't need closure. He may, and that is between him and God. For me, I don't need that toxic conversation. I choose me. I choose forgiveness and my peace. I do not need his validation, and I owe him nothing.

58

CHAPTER 8

HOW I TOOK MY FIRST STEPS TO A NEW PATH

John was my first boyfriend, and when I was still living at home, I used some of my savings so he could go to X-ray Technician school. He had also gotten his GED, and I wanted John to make something of his life. I really wanted him to have some of the money I saved. So, I went to my parents and said, "I want to give John the money he needs for school." My mom and I had this whole long talk about it. I told her that he had no idea I was doing this. We had a conversation, and from that talk, I knew that I *had* to help him. Ultimately, she and Steven agreed to let me help him with some of the money I had in a savings account. I told John, "This is for you. I want you to make something of yourself with it. I don't want anything from it. I want you to have a future and go to school." John's face was one of shock and happiness. He was very grateful. At first, he asked if, I was sure. He couldn't believe that I was giving him so much money. I told him that no wasn't an option. He had to take it, and I had every confidence that he would make something of himself with it.

John is intelligent, very bright, with so much potential, but he was also dealt a bum deck. He had similar burdens placed on him that were definitely not his to carry. I wasn't sure how that affected him entirely because he internalized a lot. But he wanted more for himself. I do not doubt that. I just don't think he knew how to get his life started, and a part of me does feel that for a long time, his path was written. He would go down a similar dark path as those in his family. No way should that happen. As much as he tried to hide it, he had a lot of light in him, and to me, this was how he began the first chapter of his life. He needed to know that he had potential and that someone believed in him. And I did and still do, even to this day.

Later, after my overdose experience, I was dating Jeremy, and John called me up. "I want to see you," he said. "I have something to give to you." This was sometime later, and I had no idea what he wanted. We met up, and he handed me an envelope. He wanted to pay me back the money I had given him, which had allowed him to go to school. I told him, "No, I don't want the money back." He had gotten his degree to be an X-ray tech, and he wanted to encourage me to do something with my life now. Through the years, he and I spoke and touched base often. I was very proud of him. Doing what he did opened so many doors, and his brother followed in his footsteps. John and I spoke for a while about his life, the money, and I refused it. I appreciated the thought and gesture. This reassured me about his character. I knew the man he was, and this is something many would not do.

But the universe had other ideas about this meet-up, and I guess timing is everything. Because he said, "You know, you should really do an ultrasound. It's a great field with lots of job openings and good money. You could use this money for *your* education now." John definitely was my first love. I knew that though he and I would not be together, we were meant to be positive catalysts in each other's lives. Perhaps soulmates of some kind? This conversation was written in the stars because I was working all sorts of jobs around this time; selling cars at used and new dealerships, a shot girl, waitressing… whatever I could do to make money legally. I was also at a point in my life where I was starting to feel like I didn't fit in where I was. That's kind of how things began to unravel.

After that conversation, it was like the universe was conspiring to *make* me get my act together, using someone I loved very much and had a soft spot for to get the message across. Suddenly and totally randomly, I was getting things in the mail for Keiser University for ultrasound education. Fliers with no name addressed, just stated, "resident" of the address... *Alright, wait a minute. Is someone messing with me?* I thought. That was when I really started paying attention to the universe. I would always see the number 11:11 everywhere and would experience these spiritual signs. My whole life I had always experienced signs from the universe. Though coincidental more often than not, but after John and I spoke... it ramped up. I would look at my clock, and it would be 11:11 every time. I would drive down a street, and it would be pitch dark, and the next thing you know, a streetlight would suddenly come on. If, for some odd reason, I were delayed in trying to leave my house, there was always a massive accident that happened at the same time on the road I would have had to take to get where I was going. Still, to this day, these things occur. It was as if the universe delayed me from going down that street. I used to get anxious about being late and seeing some of these signs. But now, after seeing the pattern, I just go with the flow. I do not fight the universe anymore. Even to this day, if something persistently shows up, I listen. It has never steered me wrong. I am so glad that I have, too, because if I waited on myself to have confidence or be in the "place" I wanted, I probably wouldn't have accomplished much. I have come to realize that "our" timetable may not be the "right" timetable, and whether or not we wholly understand the reasoning but the universe, God definitely knows what we need. We are shown the next steps, even if we do not understand or if it does not show itself in the way we want, that doesn't negate the fact that the next steps are revealed. Many times, we do not understand the reasoning until the lesson is learned. There is always something positive in the negative.

My mom has some psychic abilities, though I don't think she admits to it entirely. Her mother definitely did as well. She would hold objects and be able to tell things about the object or the owner of it. My mom has that too, but she doesn't utilize it as much. For those who don't believe, I challenge you to be open to the possibility that in this vast universe, we are just a speck, the beautiful intricacies are incredibly complex, and *everything* is energy. Look into quantum physics. It will open your mind to a whole new perspective. I refer to the universe as that because I believe that we are too mortal to understand the depths of it. I believe there is something we only have an idea about. Whoever or whatever you believe, whatever your religion, ultimately, the underlying tone is the same. We came from something pretty remarkable. In that, if you're willing, set ego aside, and the path will be shown to you. When referring to "ego", I do not imply just the boasting ego. But rather than making "it" all about you, shift perspective. See the larger picture. Everything is interconnected. Let go of controlling the outcomes and trust. See the positive through the negative, which is incredibly difficult to do because oftentimes the situation that is creating the distraction is very emotional. Feel what needs to be and then step back, look at it from a bird's eye view. More often than not, you will see the greater purpose for it. Apply this to all things and you will see that mindset and perspectives will change.

Speaking of the universe, I decided to finally listen to it. The signs were relentless. The fliers from Keiser kept coming, in the mail, on the floor, on a message board, literally everywhere. Random people I had met either had just had an ultrasound done or were an ultrasound tech. So, I sucked it up, feeling all sorts of insecure and completely out of place, and I signed up. I figured those signs would keep coming louder, so I figured, let's do it! Here we go! The day that I was going to take the entrance exam, I literally threw up about six times on the way there, but I did take the test, passed it, and got in. I was still working a full-time and a part-time job while trying to do school full-time. My grandmother, Arlene, told me, "Nicole, you're going to burn the candle wick at both ends." I had no idea what that really meant, but I thought, *oh, I got this.* I told her, "It's fine." I completed the prerequisites and was accepted into the program... continuing to think I knew best. Grandma kept telling me to slow it down... I thought I had it all under control. Well, she was right. I ended up failing out.

I had to wait three months for the course to come back around. And I did. Dean Moore was probably another universal trigger, because Dean Moore was the catalyst for the next part of my story. At the time, I had earned a variety of letters. Some A's, B's, and C's. Then that D. It was an eye sore on my transcript. Every time I thought about it, I got a bit teary-eyed. It was like a glaring reminder of my GED and other failures. I couldn't wrap my head around it. I was working two jobs, going to school, and got that D. The significance of it I really did not understand until much later.

I started ultrasound school again, and by this time, I had moved in with my grandmother, Arlene. At the time, she was living in Sunrise, Florida, and Jeremy and I had broken up. He and his sister had made a mess of my credit, so I was done with all that. It was so bad that I had to choose my credit or my future. One was interlocked with the other, but which was more important? They cleaned out my savings and ran up a few credit cards, all before I was 21 years old. All I wanted was to "just get my life started." I was not going to repeat the past mistakes. So, I considered stopping working, moving in with grandma, and letting the credit go to crap. The way I saw it then was I had to focus. I couldn't fix the credit without a future. I had to invest in myself.

When I failed out, Dean Moore told my grandma, with me sitting there in her office, that because I was going on academic probation, she had her doubts about me. She told me that maybe I should choose something "easier." She didn't think I was "smart enough" to be able to handle the ultrasound program. I was so annoyed. I was so angry. Who are you to say these things? You don't even know me. Wow! Oh boy, was I lit. What a fire that sparked in me. That solidified the decision. I quit working, lived with grandma, and waited out those three months. I look back now and think that

had to be something that the universe wanted me to hear so that
fire in my soul would light and prove her wrong.

64

CHAPTER 9

TRY, TRY, AND TRY... TILL IT STICKS

I waited my three months for the course to come back around and joined one of the classes in progress. I was doing well. Focused. Learning. Earning A's. Once again, the universe was about to test me. The mean girls came out of the woodwork. I was a people pleaser; there was no denying that. I wanted friends. True friends. I wanted to fit in. To be seen. I met a person named Joy. She was odd for sure. She would always say outlandish things and was a pathological liar. But somehow, she and I got along. We had a little group of us that would study, do lab together, and I finally felt like I fit in. Next thing I knew, I was being singled out in class and no partners to work with in the labs. I didn't understand. I kept a low profile, tried to minimize any drama, and maintain professionalism. This went on for weeks. It was actually starting to play with my mind.

One random day, I saw our class president, Michelle, in the restroom. I asked her what was up. Now this was hard for me, because remember I don't like conflict. She explained to me that Joy had been going around behind my back, telling my classmates that I was partying instead of studying. Wait. What? I was always down for a party back then, but not with all this on the line. This came about because one day, I happened to miss school because I had pneumonia, and so did three others in our group. Joy saw this as an advantage and told everyone we were skipping class to be at the beach. "I don't understand what's going on," I said. "I was out sick." I was not close with Michelle to tell her all my business, but I was definitely not partying. Nor did I want to risk anything or get involved with drama that would set me back.

Michelle said she believed me and then asked, "Can you speak with her? Ask her why she did this with some of us in the class present?" The class president totally set me up. I had no idea at the time. All I could think was that I wanted to clear my name. "You should talk to Joy with all of us present. Maybe that way we can sort this out," she pressed on. The professors, the deans, and the program directors all knew I was being singled out. This had gone on for weeks. Nothing changed. Joy continued to lie, and I continued to get picked on. So, this idea that Michelle had thrown out seemed like a potential way to solve the bullying.

I spoke with my girlfriend, Irina, who is Russian, and let her know what was going on. She couldn't believe it. She also agreed to the idea Michelle had. At this time, I still had no real control over my emotions, and it was one extreme or the other. Either a carpet to walk on, or this rage, but not in a way that was harmful to others. It was just this explosion of emotions because I had suppressed them for so long. With this going on and the idea Michelle brought up, I knew there would be potential for losing my cool. Irina was tough. We were friends and I respected her. She could totally kick my ass. Hands down. So I asked her to be present and said, "Whatever you do, don't let me hit her," I begged. "I do not want to be thrown out of the program. Please."

Irina had a temper, and that Russian fire too. She agreed not let me lose it. She went with me to be there while I engaged in this conversation. We met in the "courtyard," and the class was there. Looking back, and sitting here writing this, I can't believe how naive I was. But I was. I confronted Joy and asked her why she was lying to the class about me. Joy said something stupid that I don't really remember, but I do remember looking at her and wanting to do something rash. Here I am trying to get everything in my life together, and she is lying about it. I am not even sure why. I thought we were friends. The conversation went in circles. She was lying through her teeth, and I called it out at every turn. I felt my heart racing, and my mouth got dry. I took a breath, looked Joy in the eye, and said, "You know what? At least I can sleep at night. I'm not sure about your conscience." I turned around, took a few steps away from her, and I thought I was done. And then something in me snapped. I have no idea what happened, but I could not let her do these things and say these things. Rationale was out the window at this point. She was wrong and making up all these lies, and I needed to stick up for myself. So, I spun back around and spit right in Joy's eye. To this day, I'm not even sorry for doing it. She deserved it. I didn't hit her. But, I did show her as the trash I thought she was for all she had done. Lies. Bullying. Gaslighting. Defamation. Slander. Harassment. She was doing all of those things, and for what reason, I am not sure. In my mind, I knew exactly what came next. I went right upstairs to Dean Moore's office and told her what had happened.

The crazy part is, I had gone to the school multiple times about the bullying, and it was just brushed off. I went several times for weeks looking for help. Nothing came of it. I took full responsibility for my actions, but Joy had it coming. I just hoped I hadn't blown a chance on my future as a result. I am not really sure what test the universe was offering. Self-love? Accountability? Walking away? Not allowing it to bother me? I chose self-love. I tried the "right way," but it fell on deaf ears.

Well, once again... I got kicked out. I had to wait three months again, come back, and at that point, Dean Moore basically told me I was a lost cause. She continued to insist that I would never amount to anything. I still have no idea how a dean speaks this way to students. But she was not going to be defining my life. At that time, you had three chances to make it through the program, so I waited my time and re-entered class number three where I left off. Third time's a charm, right? I was making it through. Nothing was going to take me off course. Especially not Dean Moore.

Less than a year later, it was all worth it to see the look on Dean Moore's face when she had to pin me at graduation for being valedictorian, top of my graduating class. On my transcript, you see a variety of A's, B's, C's, and *the* **D**, followed by straight A's through the master's degree. The harder it got, the better I did. My class picked me to speak at graduation. I graduated with academic honors, made the Dean's list, and more. All of that was amazing. I needed to be pinched. Never would I have thought the D and Negative Nelly Dean Moore would be my catalysts. I was never going to give my power away to them. Not to Dean Moore, not to Joy, and not to any obstacle that came my way.

I dictate my future. I call the shots, and I will become everything they thought I wouldn't. Their negativity led to so much positivity. I am forever grateful to have encountered them. They were one of my toughest hurdles, and I leaped way over it.

Returning to school for my PA education during undergrad and within the program, Dean Moore's voice was in my head. As a result, I received straight A's the majority of the time. I graduated from Barry University with a 3.9 and the PA program with high honors, was inducted into Pi Alpha, and won multiple awards during my undergraduate and graduate stay. True, there were other factors at play, but she was a significant part of it. I could have chosen to listen to her, especially since her theme was the same as I thought everyone else's was. I refused to believe it. Little did I know how impactful her comment and my response to it would be. She was the final straw in this negativity. People thought that the circumstances that were beyond my control were going to dictate my future. Well, I was not going to allow that. I was beginning to see that we are not defined by what has happened to us but by how we handle it. I was not going to give in. I was going to be the apple that went far away from the tree.

I loved being a sonographer. The vast majority of people do not realize what we learn and what we do. It's so much more than "taking pictures." We have to learn the anatomy and physiology of adults, pediatrics, neonatal care, and obstetrics, as well as fetal development and so much more. Ultrasound education is built on physics, anatomy, and physiology. Extensively. To give you an idea, if you imagine the liver, for example, we learn about the anatomy (segments, biliary system etc.), hormones and its effects on other organs, normal and abnormal measurements of the bile ducts, pathology present and its effects on the organ and other organ systems. Or with fetal anatomy, the circulation is completely different from neonatal or pediatric circulation. Which ducts close, what happens if they don't, effects of that, measurements of all the fetal bones at the various weeks of gestation (normal and abnormal), the pathology associated with it, and how that affects development and physiology. We learn about all the pathologies and diseases that affect every age and stage of life and at conception. Earning my associates degree as a sonographer tested me in so many ways with my confidence, self-love, and facilitating the rebuilding of my foundation. One with its own purpose that had yet to be discovered.

Despite failing my ultrasound boards twice before becoming credentialed, I have earned nearly all specialties to be credentialed over the years, and was a clinical preceptor. I also gained some pretty incredible experiences in trauma, research, high-risk obstetrics, musculoskeletal, a vast array of procedures, and cardiac. I worked as an ultrasound tech for some time, and while I love the anatomy, pathology, and pathophysiology of it, after years of the same routine, I started to get bored. It became too routine. I was feeling that "tug" that I *needed* to do something else. I just was not sure what that was. Little did I know my career as a sonographer was preparing me for something else. A beautiful foundation to build upon.

GALVANIZING CLARITY

Just before I hit my 10-year mark as a sonographer, my girlfriend, Angela, who was working with me, brought up the idea of being a Physician Assistant, now titled Physician Associate (PA). I had no idea what this was, and I was intrigued. She was planning to do this. I looked into it and thought, *This is pretty cool. Maybe I could do this too.* But then I went back into those negative comments I had for myself. *I got a GED. I'm a dropout. I'm not smart enough for this.* I went down those rabbit holes for a bit. I was incredibly hesitant to potentially leave a career that I fought so hard for to jump into the unknown. I didn't want a repeat. The negative comments again popped in, but thankfully, I was able to drown them out faster this time. I saw how far I came. I saw the obstacles I hurdled over. Well, after tripping on them a few times. So I let the idea of it sit. Let's see how this comes out. Any decision to be made must be based on logic, reason, not bias and emotion. So, I waited.

I am grateful for my time as a sonographer. Working with the institutions I had and learning from some pretty amazing staff contributed to who I am now. I have learned so much from everyone. Several physicians supported me and kicked me in the ass to make me go further. One of them really lit the fire. That was Dr. "A". It was unexpected for sure. Dr. "A" and I had a patient together one night, where he ordered a sonogram. If you remember, as a sonographer, we learn labs and imaging as well. We have to be familiar, so we know what we are looking for. I asked him some questions and commented on the eosinophilia the patient had. Elevation of these labs with other supporting information can indicate a possible parasitic infection. After I commented, he just kind of looked at me strangely, with surprise and intrigue. I brushed it off and did the exam. It was maybe a month or so after that when he said, "I need to talk to you." I felt like I was in trouble. I have to admit, when I hear those words or similar, I feel like I'm getting called to the principal's office. *Oh, shit. What did I do?* I thought.

To my surprise, the first words out of his mouth were, "Nicole, you need to go to med school." I didn't even know what to say to this man. I stood there looking at him in shock, not believing that was what he had said. I am not one for a loss for words; however, I just stood there, looking at him. "I will pay for you to take the MCAT," he continued. "But you need to go to med school. You're made for more than ultrasound." He went on to remind me about that patient I had spoken up about. "What you said about that patient... You were right, and you need to move forward in your career." Still, I just stood there, shocked. He was adamant. I could not believe what I was hearing for so many reasons. Especially because while I knew him professionally, I was not close with him like I was with some of the other physicians. I also was not used to taking compliments. Quite honestly, it still can be awkward, but I'm learning.

That was a movie moment. He was the "angel" who brought the idea to life. He was the catalyst. The ripple in the pond if you may. Here was a physician I respected, but did not know well, who pulled me aside to tell me something he saw in me. For sure, this had to be a universal implant. His words stayed with me. I couldn't stop thinking about it. I definitely did not think I was smart enough for medical school. Plus, I was "too old" to be starting over, or so I thought.

Finally, I was starting to recognize that the universe was putting people in my life to trigger me to do big things, even though I did not have confidence in myself. This was becoming a pattern I couldn't ignore. Trust me, I tried. I procrastinated. But I just kept thinking this man felt so strongly about what I should do that I had to take note of that and act on it. Plus, these signs kept coming at me. It will do that. Smack you right in the face until you make the move. It begins subtle, and then so visible you cannot refuse it. I had to listen. Confident or not, it was time to move. This unusual scenario in addition to two other physicians who had no idea what Dr. "A" said, supported his thoughts. One let me know that I had an innate instinct, and a talent coupled with gestalt that takes years to develop. He strongly encouraged me to go to medical school as well. GED to Dr.? Woah, now that was a concept. These conversations came about 20 years before I actually earned my doctorate as a PA.

What I did notice was that throughout my career as a sonographer, I encountered drama. Not just the regular work things, but personal attacks on who I was and things I said. This theme is not new, but it was getting tiring. One example was when I was working at a diagnostic center in Broward County. The techs there back scanned everything I did. This is not particularly unusual, at least at that time, because you need to be proficient and know what you're doing. We manage the probe and have to know the physics of the machine. So, it was not the back scanning that was the issue; usually, the most experienced tech or manager would often the radiologists too. That was okay. It is part of the profession, and in my humble opinion, should be especially so with new graduates. You need to earn the trust. It, same in life, is not just given. The radiologists need to trust the sonographer. The problem was that they deleted my images and submitted things that were not mine as mine. I caught two of the girls doing just that, and they thought I would expose them. So, I guess they decided to set me up.

One afternoon, at the same diagnostic center, I was having a conversation with one of the radiologists about a spelling bee. I am not talking on a national level, just at primary school. I had won first place one year in grade school. This came up because someone he knew had gone national. During the conversation, one of the girls (same one I caught deleting my images) came up, interjected, and accused me of lying. It was the weirdest thing. I thought, *I just met you. Why would you do that?* Think of what she did as a conversational photobomb. I was confused. The next day, I was let go from my job. It was probably for the best because I didn't want to be in an environment like that, and I moved on to bigger and better things.

When the idea of becoming a PA came around, there was some turmoil at work with one of the supervising techs, making things very unpleasant there. I didn't know then, but I believe things were occurring, making it uncomfortable so that I would make a change, again. Every time it was time to level up, drama preceded it, making me feel uneasy and leading me to make the change. The choice was to stay in routine in what I had outgrown or step into the unknown, into possibility. While I am not one for change, I do know that it is necessary for growth. So, I jumped forward, eyes squeezed tight, fingers crossed, and praying that it would all work out. Making huge changes on faith and possibility is scary. From every aspect. Financially, emotionally… *but, PA, here I come!*

First, I had to complete my bachelor's degree *and* be in the top 10% of my class to be accepted. I needed to stand out among thousands of applications. Andrew, who is now my husband, was supportive of the idea of my going back to school. I had to include him in the process because if he wanted to be a part of my life, he had to know what he was getting himself into. I needed to be fair to him. He would go from being center stage in my life to a few steps down because school had to trump everything. I *needed* to get in, and the PA program acceptance is just as difficult, if not more difficult, than medical school because of increased demand to get into the program.

For those who do not know, a PA is an extension of the physician. There are too many patients and definitely not enough physicians. There are multiple reasons for this. The specialization of medicine is largely a contributing factor, with increased demand and a lack of residencies. Regardless, I had to focus, not only on dealing with my own insecurities and making up for past mistakes, but also on processing my past traumas with education and the challenges that came with it. I now needed to learn the foundation and associated information to be able to take care of my future patients. The programs are very demanding. We learn a large percentage of what the physicians do in 24-27 months, depending on the program. So, if you imagine our first year is equivalent to four years of medical school. Our second year is four years of residency in that short timeframe. We are trained on the medical model and trained in all the core specialties alongside physicians. When we graduate, we take a national certifying board and apply for our state medical license in addition to our prescribing license for general medications and the optional controlled substance license. There are residencies as well, in many specialties. Overall, we are ready to go into most specialties at the time of graduation. Of course, with anything, there are always things to learn, but more often than not, we can take off running with our collaborating physicians. PAs have become valued members of the team, especially with the changing needs of the patients and medicine.

Additionally, PAs learn" battlefield medicine," correlating to its origin. PAs came about to expand access to healthcare in the mid-1960s. Our original name was physician associate, and there are a handful of programs that utilized this name even after it was renamed physician assistant. Recently, our original name was returned and went back from "assistant" to "associate." The first graduating class was in 1967 from Duke University. A cardiologist who was renowned in his field for groundbreaking cardiovascular research saw that physicians were overwhelmed with the large number of patients and the shortage of physicians in primary care, which is worse now. In 1965, he put together the first class comprised of four Navy corpsmen. The men were taught medicine based on "his knowledge of the fast-tracked training of doctors during World War II," as stated by AAPA. The goal was to fill the gap and increase access to patients due to the shortage of physicians. So, you can imagine how intense the programs are, which is why I needed to be fair to my then-boyfriend, now husband. If I were going to finish the bachelor's and begin another two and a half years, I wanted him to be aware of the challenges ahead. Five years is a lot to give up. If he wanted something different, I wanted to give him the option beforehand to leave or stay.

I remember telling him, "I need to let you know that this is going to be demanding, taking a lot of my time, and you are probably going to go from being first and second in my life list to last. I want to give you an out now, because of how I am. When I go all in on something like this, there's no turning back. I'd love for you to stay, but if you don't want to, or think it will be too much, I understand, and you can leave if you would like."

I had an idea of the work that was coming, and I knew that my trauma bond from the past was absolutely going to affect my behavior, because I was *not* going to repeat the past. Failure and not getting in were not an option. My intensity level was the total opposite this time. He looked at me like I was the biggest asshole ever when I said that to him. I don't think he fully grasped what all this entailed until I was actually in it. But for some reason, he didn't walk out. I know it seems that I was being mean, but I wanted to be fair to him, considerate of his feelings and what he wanted for himself. I did not want him to look back and resent me for anything. Granted, I was doing this for us, but it was for me more than anything. No one can take my education from me. Plus, it was a way to help others on a larger scale.

Life brings all sorts of things. It is beautiful and cruel at the same time. I had become used to people leaving my life, and while he chose to stay then, there was no guarantee. Life could move us in different directions, and I never wanted to be fully dependent on another. My education is mine. But if anybody deserves a star, that man does, because he has put up with my shit and, through it all, he has been incredibly supportive. Don't get me wrong, we went through some really challenging times. A few times I didn't think our relationship would survive; we overcame many challenges, drifted apart for several years, but he remained steadfast, and he has no idea how much that means to me.

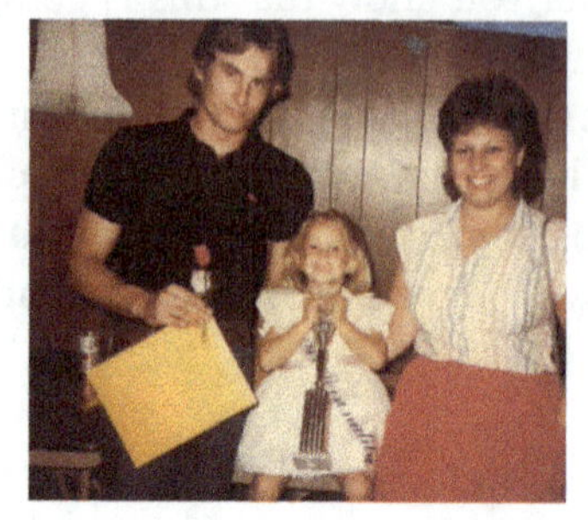

Miss Cinderella Pageant

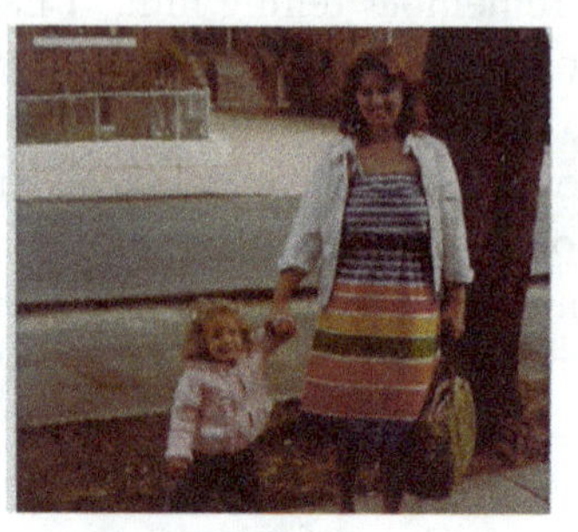

*Nicole and Mom, 1982,
around the adoption time*

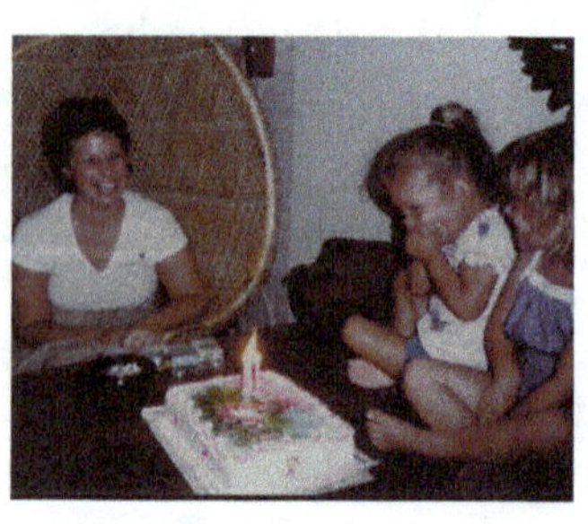

Nicole, 1983 three years old

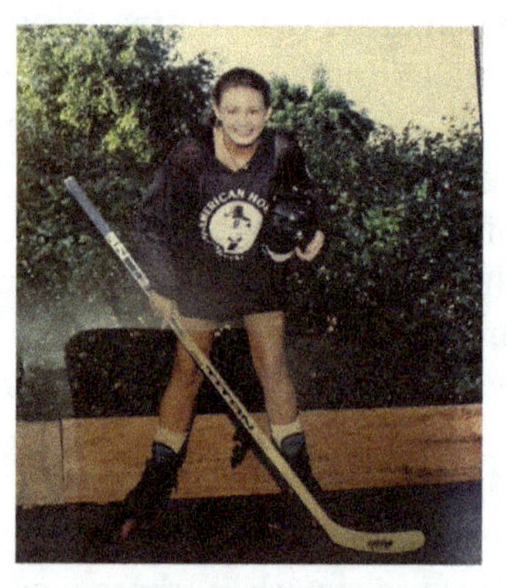

Nicole Hockey Days

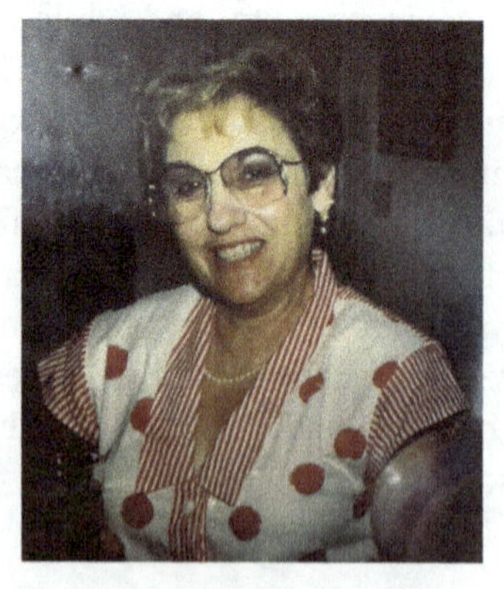

Grandma Arlene

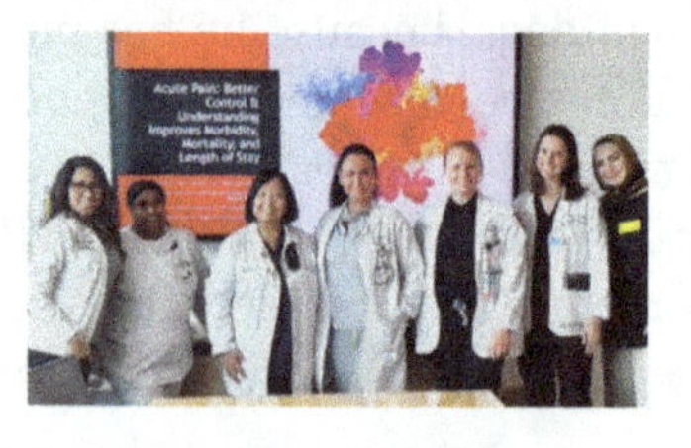

*Acute pain lecture
for nursing staff*

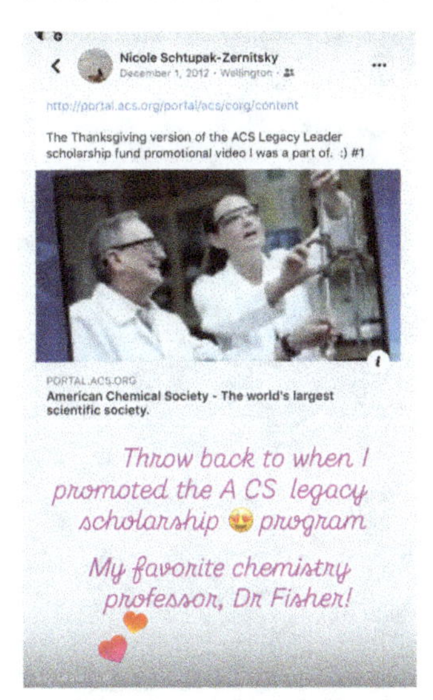

ACS Legacy Leader Scholarship for the American Chemical Society. Chosen as part of a campaign for this scholarship program

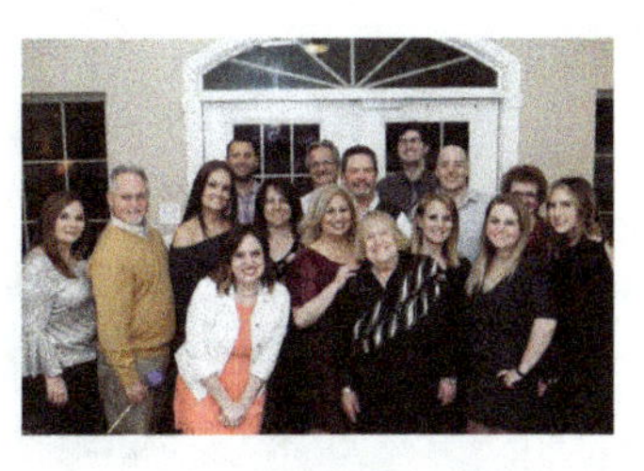

Family

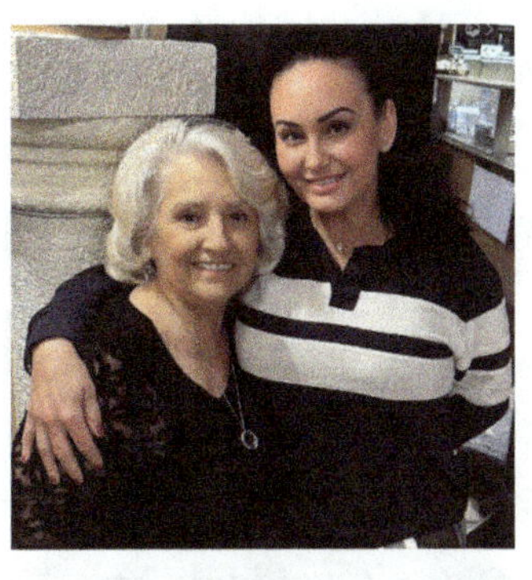

Aunt Lorraine and me

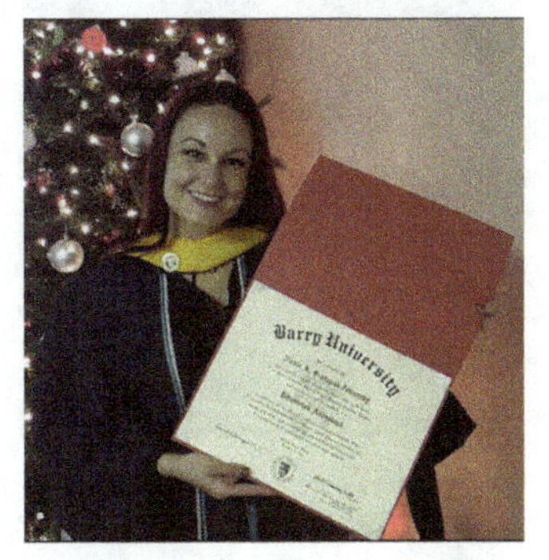

Bachelor of Science degree, graduated summa cum laude, and won several awards

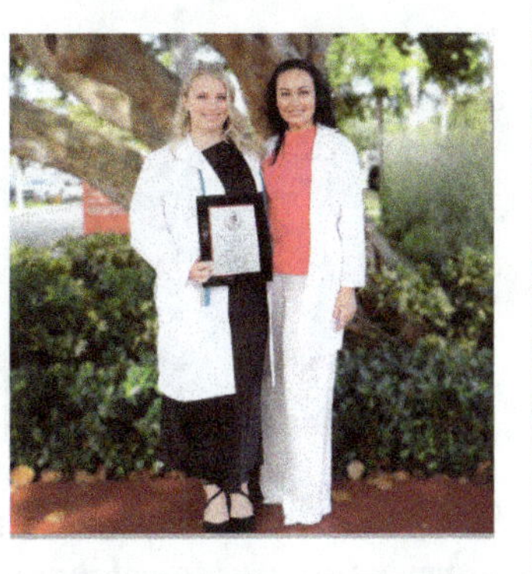

Brit and me at her PA School graduation

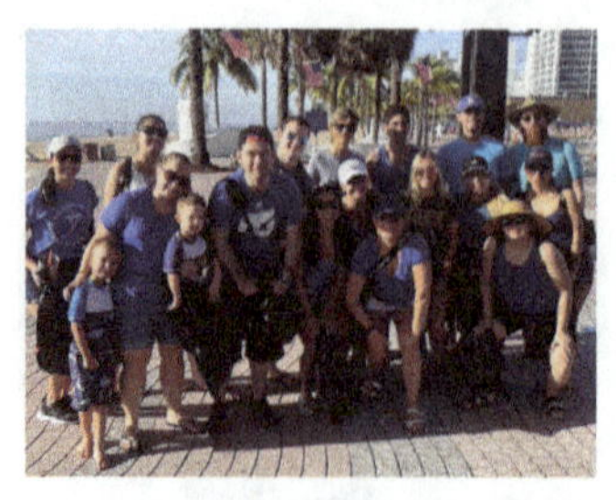

Dominican Republic Medical Mission trip

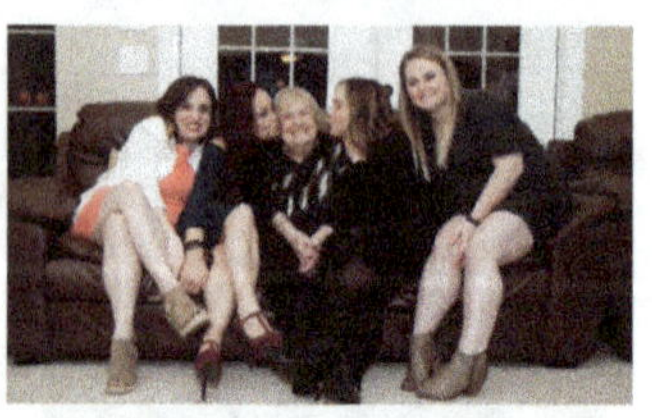

Grandma Evelyn and the Oldest Granddaughters at Mom and Bill's Wedding

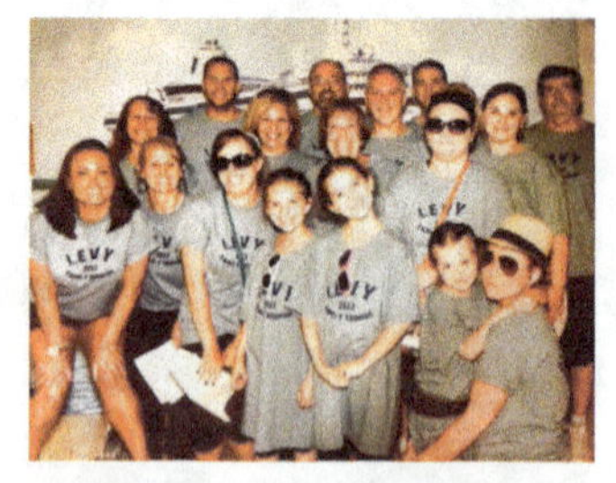

Family cruise after Grandpa Larry's passing to celebrate what would have been their 50th wedding anniversary

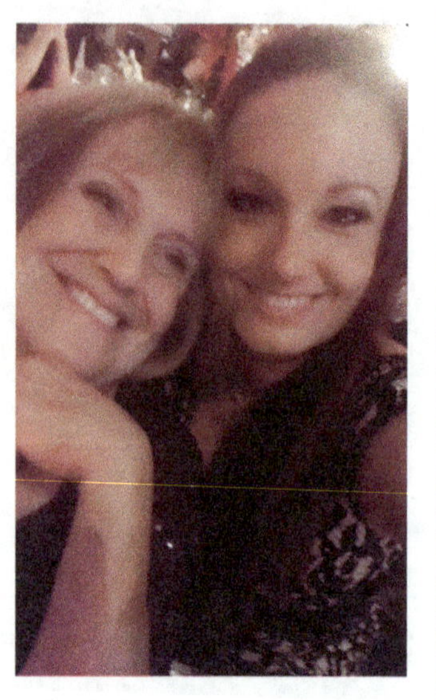

Grandma Evelyn and me

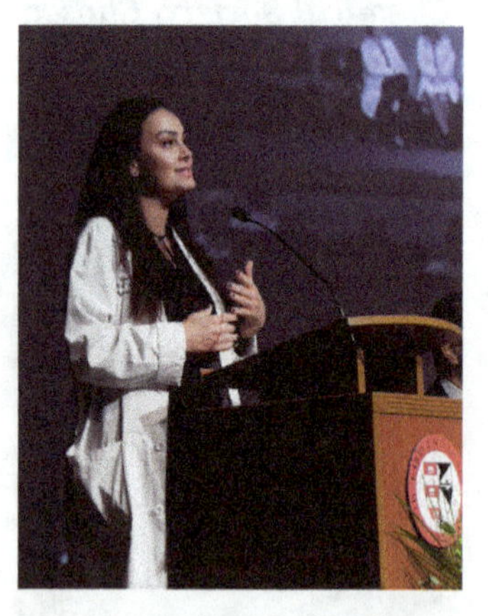

Students elected me as the keynote speaker for 2024 and 2025 at the Barry University PA Program Graduations

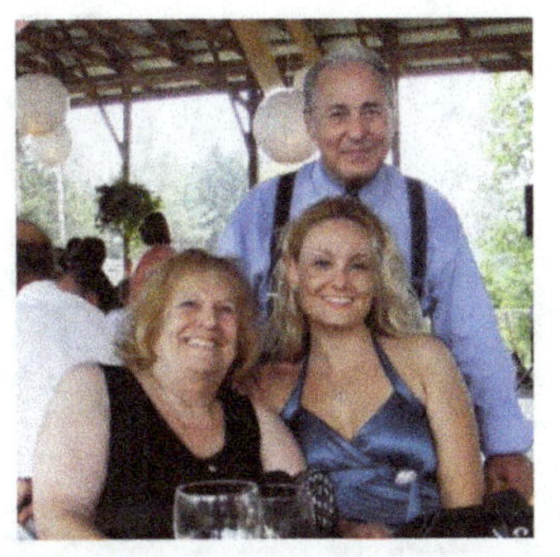

Grandma Evelyn, Grandpa Larry, and me at Uncle Jackie's Wedding

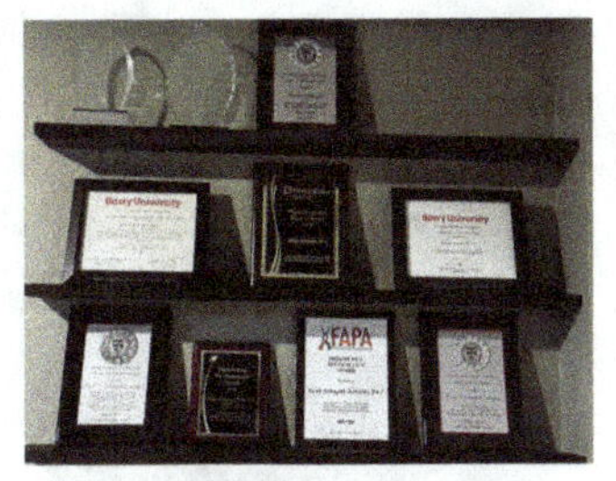

Multiple Awards over the years

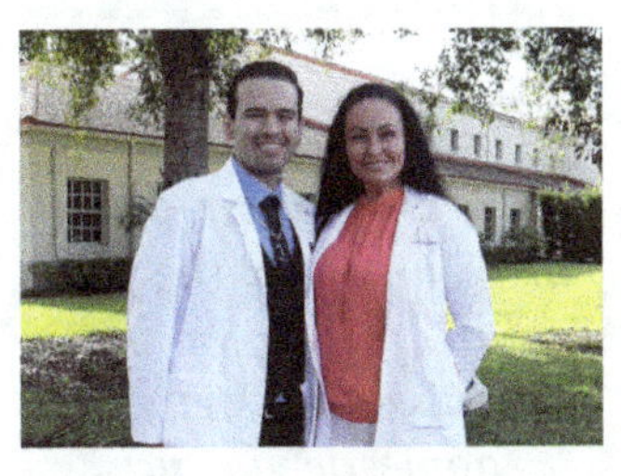

Me with Johnny, one of my students, at his graduation

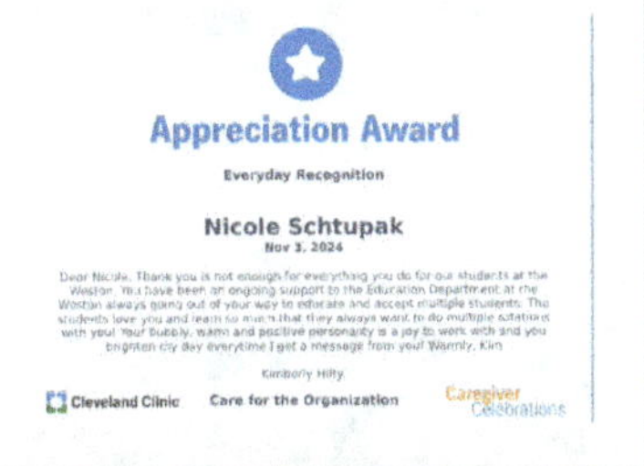

Recognition for precepting students

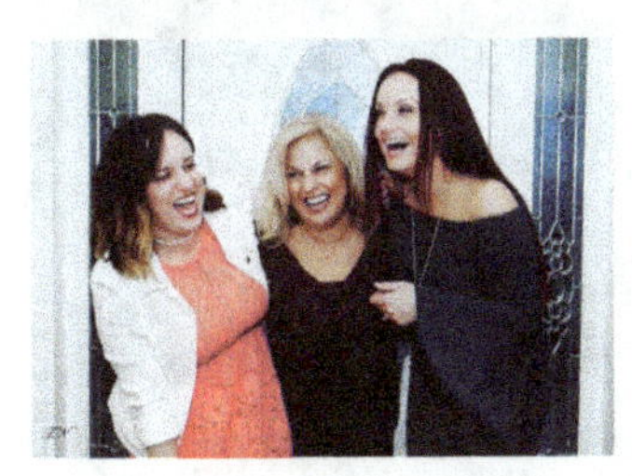

Mom Sam, and I at Mom and Bill's Wedding

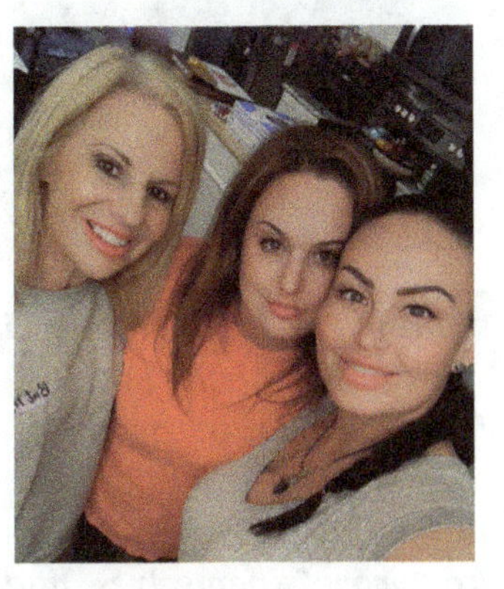

Mom, Sam and me

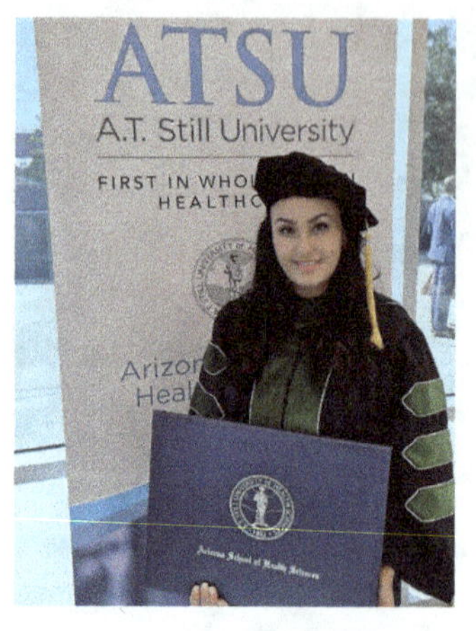

*Doctorate Graduation
from ATSU*

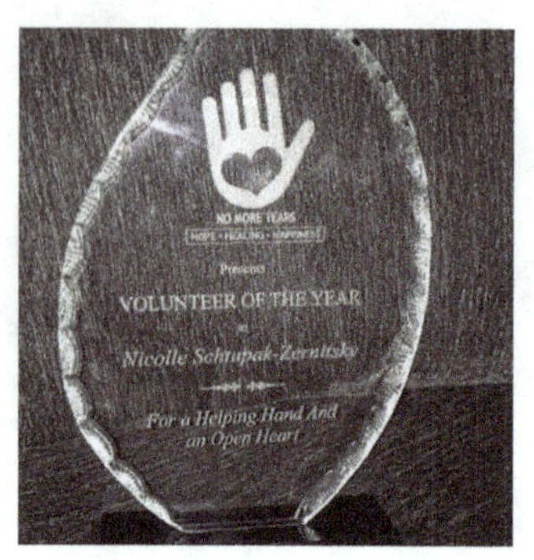

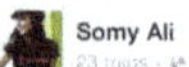

All of us at NMT would like to thank and congratulate **Nicolle Schtupak-Zernitsky** for being the volunteer of the month! Nicolle's time with NMT has been remarkably helpful. She has organized numerous events for NMT to help us raise funds.

www.nmtproject.org

*Award from non-profit
as volunteer of the year
and the month for efforts
to raise awareness for
domestic violence*

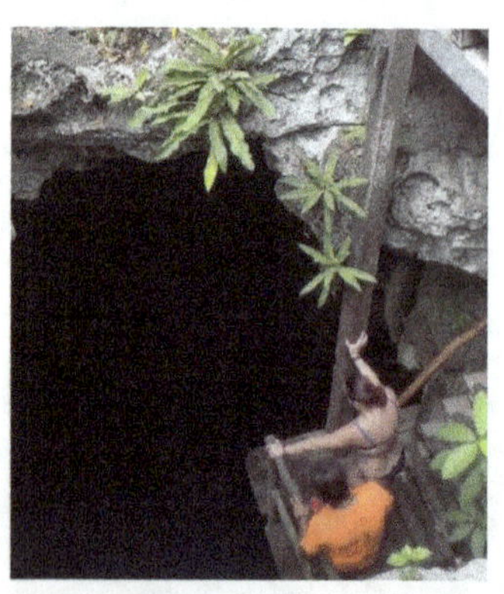

*Tulum, México. Conquered
fear of heights by jumping
from a 20foot platform into
the Cenote below. Legend
has it that Mayan warriors,
to "prove" themselves, had
to jump into this cenote.*

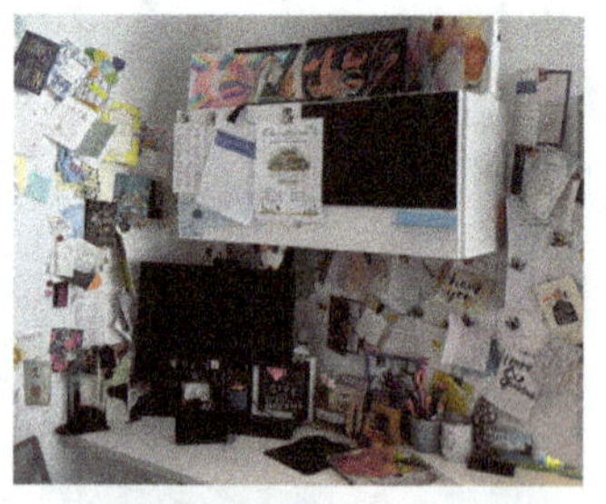

*Office With walls of
thank you cards from
students over the years*

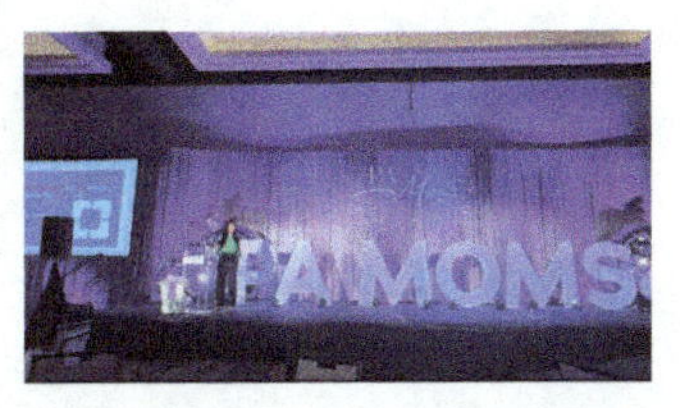

Lecturing at the PA Moms Conference in Texas, 2025

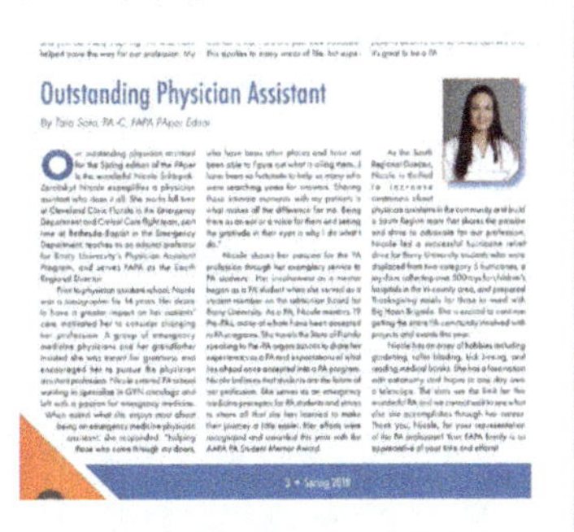

Outstanding Physician Assistant

By Tara Soto, PA-C, FAPA PAper Editor

Article in the Paper

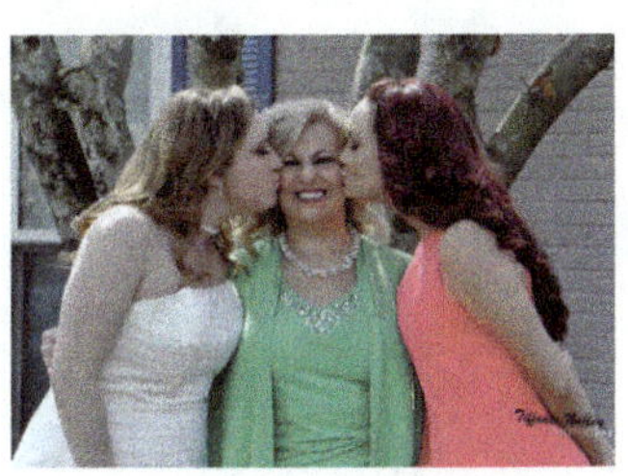

Sam, Mom, and me

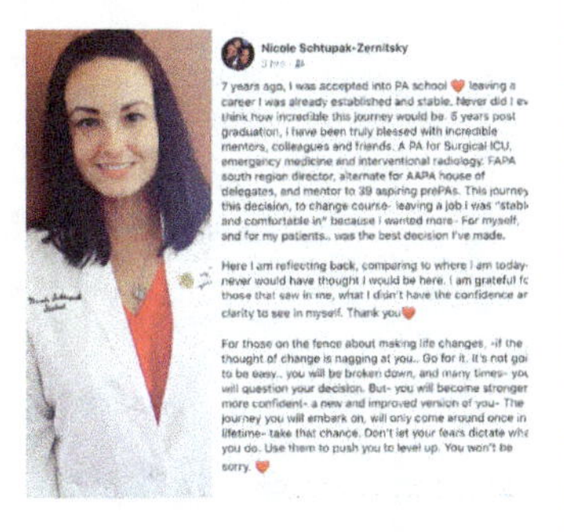

Nicole Schtupak-Zernitsky
3 hrs ·

7 years ago, I was accepted into PA school ♥ leaving a career I was already established and stable. Never did I ev think how incredible this journey would be. 5 years post graduation, I have been truly blessed with incredible mentors, colleagues and friends. A PA for Surgical ICU, emergency medicine and interventional radiology. FAPA south region director, alternate for AAPA house of delegates, and mentor to 39 aspiring prePAs. This journey this decision, to change course- leaving a job I was "stabl and comfortable in" because I wanted more- For myself, and for my patients.. was the best decision I've made.

Here I am reflecting back, comparing to where I am today- never would have thought I would be here. I am grateful fc those that saw in me, what I didn't have the confidence ar clarity to see in myself. Thank you ♥

For those on the fence about making life changes, -if the thought of change is nagging at you.. Go for it. It's not goi to be easy.. you will be broken down, and many times- you will question your decision. But- you will become stronger more confident- a new and improved version of you- The journey you will embark on, will only come around once in lifetime- take that chance. Don't let your fears dictate wha you do. Use them to push you to level up. You won't be sorry. ♥

Reflecting, after acceptance into PA School

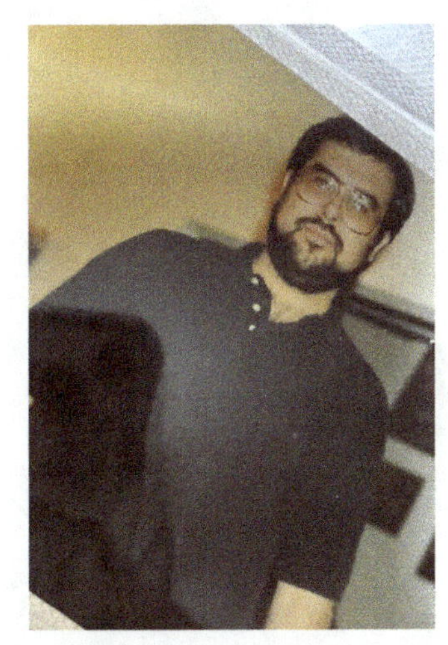

Steven Schtupak

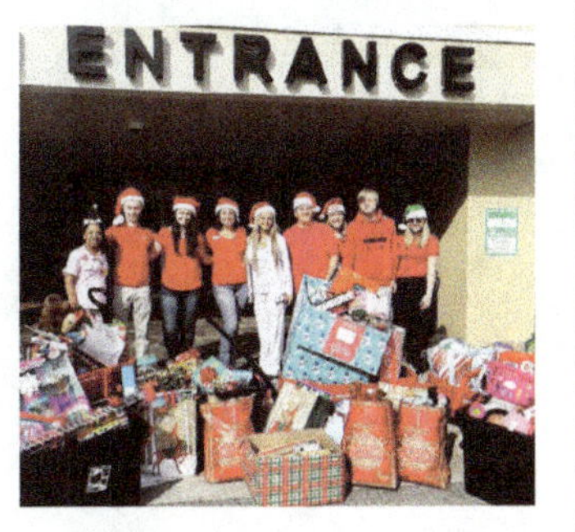

Toy Drive for the Tri-County area

CHAPTER 10

LOSING A SOULMATE – GAINING POWER FROM PAIN

Bad things happen. We lose people we love. The first person I ever lost in the sense of death, the first genuine loss, was my grandfather, Larry. He, aside from my mom, was also my biggest advocate. Mom used to call him my knight in shining armor. He was my rock, the one thing that I trusted above all else. He facilitated a better relationship between my mom and me. In my early 20s no matter how much I was trying, little wins here and there, Mom would be very negative. I guess it was a combination of things, she was unhappy, and before I began to straighten up, I gave her every reason not to trust me. What was so frustrating is that at that time, she just didn't see it. She continued to revert back to the past. In my humble opinion, I do not think she realized what she was doing. I think it was reactional from what she knew growing up. In addition to her not being happy at that time, this clouded her judgment. One day, I was so upset and venting to Grandpa that I told that man everything. He called Mom and "straightened her out." That was the tipping point, and Mom and I began to heal our relationship. Grandpa and I were always close, but our relationship deepened when I was in my early 20s. This was after my accidental overdose, and I was on a mission to get it together. This apple was going light-years away from the tree. Then, when I was younger, I had a hard time deciphering my feelings. The reason for this was multifactorial. But I didn't know how to express how I was feeling productively, lived in flight or fight mode on defense constantly. So, if I had a conflict of some sort because I did not know what an appropriate response vs. was emotional, he helped me learn how to have a voice. Grandpa and I spoke all the time, at least three to four times a week if not more. He was my best friend. Often, I would call him seeking his guidance. "Hey, this is the scenario. This is what happened. This is how I feel. Is that right?" I was so screwed up for so long that I couldn't even decipher my own feelings. Grandpa Larry was a soulmate. Hands down. I do believe we have many soulmates in this life. My mom is one, my sister is another one, and my grandfather is definitely one. Aside from the man he was, one of the things I loved most was that he knew all of the things that I was going through and loved me despite all of it. Unconditionally. He was the first person that I saw and felt love from, despite the darkness I had. He was my rock. The calm in the storm. I owe so much of who I am to him because he loved me.

For other people, I had to put on a show and pretend to be this happy, smiley person, especially with boyfriends. I remember a guy I dated when I was around 18 years old. We were at the point of discussing our families and our upbringing. I liked this guy, but definitely not in love. I was very hesitant to discuss my background. I felt like I would be judged, especially because I judged myself on it, even though I had no control over it, especially how life began for me. I tried to delay the conversation, but the point came when I could not avoid it any longer. I didn't want to tell him the truth. I was ashamed, embarrassed. I remember thinking, *do I only talk about Mom and Steven? Or do I include the biological donor and hospital stuff?* I decided to tell all the things. I reasoned that if by some chance this lasted, I did not want him to be angry with me for not telling the truth. Because to me, omission is just as bad. I let it out. A watered-down version, of course, but it was out. Well, it went south. Fast. I remember the look of shame and disgust on his face. The judgmental stare. I knew exactly what he was thinking.

And boy was I right. Literally, his next words were, "I'm sorry, but I cannot date you. You are too damaged for me."

I. Was. Mortified.

It would be years before I said anything even remotely close again. Looking back, I know now he was the problem, and I definitely dodged a bullet there. But it hurt. I felt so ashamed and embarrassed. Dirty. Undeserving. I cried for hours after. Not because of him, but his words and how he said them. It was terrible. His response was a contributing factor for me keeping men at arm's length. *Why bother getting close? If people know the real you, that is what they will think,* I thought. *Or they leave you. So what is the point,* I would think. It wasn't just men; I have kept most everyone at arm's length. Especially women. Perhaps stemming from my "mother and father wounds" and the abandonment by both my biological parents.

Grandpa was the first person who I felt loved me without the façade, and when he passed away suddenly, I felt a piece of me die. I know that sounds dramatic. But I closed off for a long time after that. Around that time, life was good. I was in school, earning the grades, learning to love and let my guard down, engaged to be married, everything was perfect. I was truly happy. The kind of happiness you have without waiting for the other shoe to drop. I was coming out of survival mode... or so I thought. The night he passed was awful. We had spoken a few days prior, and all things were "right with the universe." That night, though, I couldn't sleep. My neck and back ached. I just couldn't get comfortable. I had never felt anything like that before, and no injury. I tossed and turned all night. It was awful. I took Ibuprofen, Acetaminophen, and nothing.

I was living in Coral Springs with my fiancée at the time. My grandfather was supposed to walk me down the aisle. That night—well, morning—I fell asleep at about 6:30 in the morning and then my phone started blowing up. My mom must have called me a dozen times back-to-back. Texts and calls from my uncle, my mom, and my aunt. Finally, I picked up, and Mom informed me that Grandpa had passed away. It was like a piece of me died. Grasping the phone, I cried and let out a yell that a person who is legally deaf would have heard.

The last time I had felt that strong an emotion was when I found out that I was adopted. But this was worse. I can't explain it. I felt all the life and air come from me, and I fell to the ground. I couldn't breathe, I couldn't see between the tears, and I let out another scream. The *one* person who was my rock and everything was now gone. He was not sick. He was just gone. My grandma said he sneezed really hard, like six or seven times, and then fell asleep in his recliner, where he slept often because he had a bad back. When she woke up, he had passed. He had uncontrolled diabetes and atrial fibrillation (abnormal heart rhythm that can cause strokes), and I think, because of the sneezing, which my grandma said was very forceful, that and having recently fallen, creating a head injury, may have caused his death. He was taking aspirin, but he wasn't on any anticoagulation (aspirin is an antiplatelet). I think he might have had a stroke because he sneezed so forcefully many times. With the uncontrolled diabetes, atrial fibrillation, and recent trauma, I suspect this as the possible reason for his sudden death. In the Jewish religion, we don't do autopsies, so we don't really know what actually happened. I hated it for me, but for him it was fast, and he likely had no idea what had occurred.

I was I definitely changed after that moment. I don't even know how my husband and I lasted as long as we did, because I shut completely down when Grandpa passed. I was numb. I pushed everyone away. Going through this and trying to get into PA school was awful. My emotions were all over the place. Anxiety was on high. I was not sure if it was a test to see if I would give up, but I refused to do so. I buried it, deep down, locked the feelings and emotions away because I *had* to keep moving forward. I just focused on school. I did not want to feel anything. I was so sick and tired of heartbreak, of loss. Everybody has said, "Oh, you got a 4.0, you're so smart." I always think, *maybe, but at what cost?* I lost friends, marriage was on the rocks, lost a piece of my heart… and shut off every emotion. I did not handle his death. I did not grieve. Nor did I want to. Because that meant feeling the pain. I shoved it so far down and I compartmentalized so that I wouldn't feel it. *I never wanted to feel this kind of pain again.* The one person, my heart, my soulmate, my safe place was now *gone*. Ripped from me without warning. I was so angry. Lost. I did not understand and felt like I was being punished. I know that sounds insane, but how I felt then was, *if there is a God, why would he allow this?* I felt so alone. Heartbroken. I wanted to revert back to my partying and self-destructive days. I wanted this pain gone. I didn't care how it went. It just needed to be gone. I shut down and nearly became "dark." Honestly, I think this is the first time I realized and learned how to alchemize pain. I could not wrap my head around it. I did not want to go down those dark paths like I previously had, but I was exhausted, mentally, spiritually, and physically. Everything seemed like a fight. Every situation, person, whether it was career, friends, family, sense of self, it didn't matter. I was always in fight or flight mode. I had felt, because I was doing everything "right," nothing bad should happen. I had no real understanding of the deeper transformation that needed to occur. I had a very hard time seeing anything positive in his passing.

I focused on school, but I shut everyone and everything out. I wanted to run away. Maybe I became "smart" because that's all I felt I had. I focused on my education because it was mine; no one could take that from me. I got tired of people leaving my life. I went back into survival mode. One of my students said something to me years later that lit a light bulb. We were talking about her life, and she said, "You know, people always talk about the quiet ones. Rarely does anyone check on the overachievers." It was an interesting and valid point of view. Especially from my own personal experiences. I was depressed and felt somehow that I was damaged and deserved all these "bad things." I felt her statement to the core, and I think we all need to be better at recognizing people who need help. At that time, I held on to something so tight, to the point where I buried myself in it because I didn't want to feel. I needed to be in control. After extensive introspection, I committed to myself. I got through the semester doing 21 credits, tutoring, teaching assistant for multiple chemistry and biology courses plus undergraduate research. I needed to stay distracted. I got involved with groups on campus and a part of a "Legacy Leadership" scholarship promotional video and article for the American Chemical Society to pay it forward and use the energy for positive. I distracted myself to keep myself from going dark. The rage, the heartbreak, was so much. I did not realize, though, how much I had shut myself off. I guess you can say I trauma-bonded to my career. While helping others is not a bad thing, and I became one of the best in my field, it was at the expense of myself. I thought at the time that it was all I had. I was *not* going to lose it. I graduated with high academic and scientific honors and did all these wonderful philanthropic things, but again, at what cost? I distanced myself from my husband, who honestly deserves a medal. I don't know how he put up with my ass.

When Grandpa died, I genuinely lost a huge piece of me and only recently feel like I am starting to come back. I was just figuring out my emotions on how to deal positively, rather than self-sabotage. My whole life, I have felt like I've lived in a stress-induced state, anxiously awaiting the next negative thing. Not only did this traumatize me or reactivate the trauma from infancy, but for quite some time, I felt like I didn't deserve to be happy. *Maybe it just was not in the cards for me,* I thought. For well over a decade after, I was always waiting for the other shoe to drop. I was actually scared to be happy. The way I saw it… Every time I was getting a sense of happiness, it would be taken away.

At Grandpa's funeral, we all gathered in the house. It was bittersweet, and I realized I missed those days when the whole family would come, the house packed to the gills, all of the family under one roof. The running joke in the family is that we behave like the Grizwalds. Outspoken, loud, sarcastic, but loving. Our whole family is so close. Grandpa Larry and Grandma Arlene wanted it that way. Perspective, Grandpa Larry and Grandma Arlene were married. They had my mom, Andrea, and my uncle, Michael. They divorced. Grandpa remarried my other amazing grandma, Evelyn. They had my Aunt Donna and Aunt Laura. They remained married until his passing. Grandma Arlene remarried to Grandpa Dick. They were married until Grandma's passing. Arlene and Larry wanted all of us to be one family. It clearly was not that easy especially in the beginning after they divorced. But what those two did by keeping us all together, revealed to me over the years as I let my guard down, is so rare. It was and is something special. I love my family so much. I could not have been luckier to be chosen to be a part of them. Oftentimes, I will feel some remorse for shutting down. Be it from my feeling like the black sheep or after Grandpa passed. They never retreated, even in my dark moments. What I love most about what my grandparents did for us all is to make us feel comfortable with speaking our mind. Saying whatever it is you need to and move on. That's exactly what we did. No grudges, no hate, none of that drama. Even if the other person doesn't like it, too bad. We hashed it out and two seconds later we were laughing. We moved on to the next moment.

For the first quarter of my life, I carried a burden that was not mine to carry. Looking back, I see that now, contrary to what Mom has told me. God never made a mistake. This was the plan. I needed them in order for me to become me, inspire others, feel confident in my voice, and develop a strength unlike anything I will never fully understand. It was they, my grandparents, my mom, aunts, uncle, sister, my dad Steven, and even "T," as absent as he was. I thought I would never recover after Grandpa's passing. It genuinely broke me. But his legacy, love for life, and his family lives on through me. Through them. They fostered a strength and a voice that only could have been done by them. You see, while I miss my grandpa and grandma so much, they never left. Reality is, I needed to break. I had to feel all of that pain for many reasons. First, at almost eleven years old, I shut down. Carrying the burden placed on me by actions of others, I defined my character as a result. I assumed things that were not true. Dealing with all things that eleven-year-olds do, bullying etc., smothers you. It's hard to see anything other than darkness after that. Yes, I retreated and completely shut down when he passed, but I needed to feel that, otherwise how do you grow? I see the need to break from the pain but not in a negative way. More so, breaking off the stone and ice walls I had been hiding behind as a shield. At first though, I made those walls higher, more durable, or so I thought.

Reflecting, everyone in my family played a role in the woman I have become. Each carries their own strengths that they instilled in me. I am so thankful. Grandpa's passing was not just painful. What I saw as a negative then, I now see as an act of love. Yes, I was unsure and did not know how to deal with those emotions, especially given all that occurred in my life up to then. But his love for me was so strong that it defeated death. At the funeral, walking up to the open coffin and seeing him, there was an interesting feeling. I felt a sense of calm. He looked at peace with these tortoise shell glasses on, which were *not* his. I kissed his forehead and thanked him for who he was, and I promised him I would carry his legacy forward. I would help others the way he did with me. While I shut down for many years, I never fully closed off, possibly out of guilt, thinking he would come back and lecture me. I felt I owed it to him to become my best self. What I didn't realize was that I was recharging. I was restoring my energy little by little, mentoring, volunteering in the community, and being involved in many other philanthropic events. I became a leader in my community with the goal of helping others. While the pain shut off one part of me temporarily, other parts that were closed off were coming alive again. The pain had to occur to break open whatever parts of me I locked away from infancy. I was regaining my power from the pain. Slowly, I was returning to myself and alchemizing it all.

MY EARLIEST MEMORIES

From the time my "parents" drove me to Florida and until I learned the truth of my birth, as far as I knew, everything was good. What I remember the most before the divorce was living in Boca Rio. I don't really remember living in the trailer until after the divorce. One of my only really good memories is of "T" and I gardening. He taught me how to grow all kind of things, flowers, vegetables, watermelons even, and now, all these years later, I am still into gardening. So much so that it is why I am working on my therapeutic and wellness garden at the hospital. I remember the night we left. I remember the car. I remember crying. I remember asking my mom why we were leaving daddy.

I don't have many good memories of living with him. Anything that is good, unfortunately, is overshadowed by everything bad. Once they got divorced, "T" was mostly missing in action. I seem to have blocked out most of my early memories of him before the divorce. I do remember a lot of yelling and fighting, mostly because "T" could never keep a job. I'm not really sure what the issue was with that, because he would never tell the truth. He always blamed everybody else, so I don't know what jobs he had or why he lost or quit them. Mom was always worried about money. I remember them fighting about money. They divorced, she said, because she got tired of him not being able to hold a job, tired of all the lies that he would offer as reason why this job or that one didn't work out.

Mom always kept at least one job. After the divorce, she worked three. My sister and I were never alone. We had babysitters, close family friends and family that looked after us while she worked. She did this until she met Steven, and that changed the game a little bit. Quite honestly, I am not sure Mom really knows how incredible she is. Yes, we had our fights, and they were some fights let me tell you! But I admire her. Her life was not easy either. While we are not biologically connected, I get much of my strength from her and we are a lot alike. No matter how tough it was, she never faltered. Even if she wanted to throw in the towel.

Mom and "T" had my baby sister when I was six years old. At first, I was excited about the idea having a sister when Mom told me the news. But there is a photo of me when she was finally born, and it is clear that I was not impressed. Ha! They call that expression the "Nicole face." Sort of a combination between a pout and mad face! I remember when my mom went into labor with her. It was late in at night, and I ended up going to one of the neighborhood friend's houses to be looked after. Nicky and Georgie were the two sons of the neighbors that I was friends with. The next day, I was brought over to the hospital, and we stood right in front of the window where all the babies are, where the families can view them. I turned around and said, "What the heck? What is this thing? We're bringing this home?" Ha! She was cute and although I made the Nicole face, I loved her from the first view of her tiny bald head through the window.

In the long run, I was happy to have a sister. I love my sister. She is a huge piece of my heart. My mom, my sister, and I, the three of us, are very close despite all the things and all the growth we all went through. We are each other's constants. I know Mom has a lot of regrets because she was not happy around the time that she married "T" and even later when she married Steven. She was just not happy with the place she was in her life. She carries tremendous guilt. I tell her all the time that the one thing that I wish for her is for her to let that go. There is no reason to carry all that. She doesn't talk much about it, but I know it was hard for her during her childhood. The Grandma Arlene I knew is not the same one she was. Grandma, too, had to "grow up" fast. What I have learned through observation and experience so far is that we all do the best we can with the information and things available at the time. Couple that with learned experiences, and that will dictate a lot. So, I know Mom has carried a burden that is also not hers. She, too, for most of her life, in my opinion, allowed that to dictate what she was worthy of. Choices she made, paths she went down… presumed delays…she sees as mistakes. Perhaps even failures. But I don't. I am glad she made all the choices she did, because it brought her to me. God was preparing her for me. Ha! For all the mischief and grey hairs I was going to give her. All joking aside, I do believe he was strengthening her. Providing all sorts of tests and experiences to 1., show her how resilient she is and, 2., prepare her for the rocky roads to come as she embraces being a mother and finding her own true passion.

THE FOUR ELEMENTS: EARTH, WATER, AIR, AND FIRE

I hate that she carries that guilt. But Mom will say she was miserable and may have taken some of her unhappiness out on us. The three of us fought. Some pretty rough words were exchanged on all ends. Why? Well, if anyone reading this has a daughter, you know at some point you are going to have those arguments. So part of that was true; we also were a lot alike. We are strong, independent, outspoken women with burdens we were carrying and trying to find our place in the world. My sister and I were "growing up" as it pertains to age and emotional growth, and Mom was just only discovering who she was. I am not sure what dimmed Mom's light so young, perhaps family dynamics and feeling as if she was discarded too. Remember Grandma Arlene and Grandpa Larry initially did not have a smooth breakup. I know Mom felt a certain way about it. I'm sure my uncle did too. I'm sure they carried that with them. I know because I did too. Children see everything. I do believe that situation affected her own light. So yeah, we disagreed. We said hurtful things, and she feels guilty about how she was then. Not that she treated us badly. We were never without anything. She loved us, more than she loved herself, and worked so hard to make sure we had everything we needed. I would bet that up to that time, my sister and I were her "true loves."

One of the things my sister doesn't realize, and one of the things I wish for her, is to see how special she is. Before she was even talking, putting sentences together, she was drawing. She is incredibly gifted with art, anything and everything creative. When she was in high school, one of her friends was going to apply to a special art school in the city. It was pretty strict and super hard to get into. They only took a certain number of people, and my sister applied more as a favor to this friend of hers, and she got accepted. Her friend did not. Here was this remarkable and rare opportunity being accepted into this amazing and difficult art program, and she didn't have the courage or belief in herself to take advantage of it. She didn't go.

My sister holds a lot of things in, and that's something I wish she wouldn't do. That kind of thing can lead a person to self-destruct. She holds a lot in about the divorce, about Steven, "Mum," and Becky. Steven was the only father she knew. When "T" and his new wife, Karen got together, at some point, he told Karen that Samantha wasn't his. He told Karen that Mom cheated on him, and Sam was someone else's kid. But it fits the pattern of his life, the constant lack of accountability. It was disgusting of him; who doesn't claim their own child? I know that must have affected her to some degree. In a way, I'm happy for her because she doesn't know the heartbreak of having a father like that. That gives me peace in a way that she didn't have to go through the disappointment of waiting for him to come take her someplace and not show up, the phone calls that never came, the birthdays and celebrations he didn't show up for, and always having an excuse without accountability. She had Steven, and he was a constant for her. Sure, they fought and had their issues. However, Steven was always there when it really counted and during the difficult times.

She was so young when Mom and "T" divorced. She doesn't really remember him at all. By the time she was maybe three or four, Steven was in the picture, and she had a father worth having. That relationship was very good until Mom and Steven divorced.

Sam was going through her own rough teenage years at that point. When Steven left to move back to Florida from Kentucky, I know that hurt her. More than she would outwardly admit. She felt like he abandoned her. What I know is that Steven was depressed at that time. He moved back to Florida because his father was sick here and there, and he moved back home to help him. Steven was worried about Sam, and he expressed that. He was also struggling with his own depression after the divorce, and he carried guilt for not being able to be there for Sam. He loved Mom, and while it was mutual, their divorce saddened him. He knew though, that it was best for them to split. It was just too toxic. Sam took it personally. Growing up, before and after I moved out, they were like two peas in a pod. She saw Steven a few months before he passed, and I think both of them took time for granted. They loved each other very much. Losing him, I know broke her heart.

Sam was also very close to Mary AKA "Mum" and Becky. They were like family. We knew them from when we lived in the trailer. They used to help watch Sam and me. Over the years, Sam became very close to them. Becky, who was "Mum's" daughter, we used to say was Sam's second mother. Becky passed away from ovarian cancer when Sam was in her tween years and my sister never processed that. She and Becky were incredibly close. It was a tough time for Sam. Mary was still alive for a little while, but then she got dementia and went to live with other relatives before she passed away. With Sam in Kentucky, when "Mum" got sick and passed, no one from Mary and Becky's family returned calls to Sam. In my humble opinion, I think what they did was wrong. It was selfish. Sam was so close to both of them, and they knew it. For them to disregard her and not even allow Sam to say goodbye if she chose to was wrong. I do not know if Sam knows this, but I called Tasha, Mary's granddaughter, and let them know how I felt about their lack of consideration for my sister. She too, has suffered her own set of trauma and loss. Despite all of that, she has such a huge heart and was always trying to be the peacekeeper in the family. She does not like conflict. She has not processed all the loss she has endured.

This worries me for her, because I know how internalizing can affect you. That too weighs on your esteem and self-love.

Sam lives right near my mom, 30 minutes over the river from my mom's house in Jeffersonville, Indiana. Mom and Steven moved to Louisville, Kentucky, with Sam when I was about twenty because Steven had lost his job. He did computer programming and had a brilliant mind. He had all the Microsoft certifications, built computers, programmed, and even developed some computer programs. I learned more about that man after he passed, because he was incredibly humble. He couldn't find any other job or any other work when they were living in Boca. I was out of the house at that time, and Sam was in middle school when they moved because Steven landed a good job in Louisville.

Over the years, the constant has always been us three. Through thick and thin, we are each other's constants. I have always felt that regardless of what happens, we will always be. We heal each other. Between the three of us, there are all four elements. Mom is a Scorpio, which is a water sign, Sam is a Leo, which is a Fire sign, and my signs (sun, rising, and moon) are Air and Earth. We complement each other as each of the elements of the earth does. We complete each other, no matter how blinded I was to it for many years.

CHAPTER 11

MOM, SAM, AND ME – THE MIGHTY TRIO

I'm incredibly proud of Mom and my sister. Mom put herself through undergrad, ultimately earning her master's degree as a licensed clinical social worker. Much of why Mom was not happy with herself before marrying Steven had a lot to do with only having her high school diploma. Raising two kids, she put herself through school, taking one class at a time until she finally graduated with her master's. Sam also went through her own dark years but earned her license as a certified nursing assistant (CNA), and also earning her certificate as a cosmetologist. She did not really like the CNA work. I think her creativity needed to be expressed, so getting her license to do cosmetology, I felt, was perfect. She's incredibly talented.

It was definitely not easy for any of us under any circumstances, but in the end, it was always the three of us. My sister asked me at one point why I left home. Sam was upset with me for a while that left her in what she liked to call "the yelling house." The fighting was terrible. The mean and hurtful things were said all around. No one was happy, at one point, for some time. This largely contributed to why I left.

I told her, "Sam, I was not in a good place. I was not happy. I was self-destructing. I felt lost. I felt not a part of the family at all." I don't know if she will ever fully grasp how sad and depressed, I was. She knows a lot of the story, but there are things I don't think she does or really realizes over the years. Pulling out my eyelashes and shaving eyebrows, cutting, contemplating suicide, self-destructing behavior, I *had* to leave. It truly was a matter of choosing myself. Mom and Steven were very supportive, but the environment also had toxicity, which both contributed to. I felt I added a layer of negativity, too. So, when I left, it was to choose myself and give my sister a chance to be happy. At that time, I felt like a lot of the infighting was because of me. I did not have the insight to see truly what was happening. How much each was suffering. I figured if I removed myself from the equation, it would be better for her and for me.

Sam was spoiled from every direction, from Mum and Becky. Steven and our family used to say, "You're going to be in for it, Andrea, if you keep it up like that." Sam was always the "favored child." Mom will deny this, but it was evident. Everyone knew it. She got everything she wanted and saw little discipline for her actions. I, on the other hand, was always disciplined, even if I didn't do anything to deserve it. Sam was in her bratty phase just around the time I left home. She would do shit to get me into trouble. There are stories I could tell. One I remember is something I would never think that this little asshole would have done to me. I'm not sure how old she was at the time, but our parents went to a Marlins game. We were living in Boca, and I was babysitting her, and I wanted her to go in the bath. So, this particular night, Sam's answer was firm. "No, I'm not getting in the bath." We went back and forth over and over. We had a white TV that sat on the dresser in her room. The screen was small, it had a big white outer box, and a weird little keyboard or something attached to it. When I was not letting up for her to get in the bath, Sam got mad, she shoved the whole thing off the dresser and cracked it, and guess who got in trouble for it? Me. She was tough when she wanted to be and stubborn as a mule. She would do things like that all the time. Even other family members would come to my defense.

I got back at her in my own way. Once, I tied her hands and feet together as if she were kidnapped, put her in my closet, and shut the door. She was little, six, maybe five, and I was a mean tween. Another time, we were playing hide and seek. My friend Melissa and her sister Heather were at the house. I told Sam, " I've got a great place for you to hide." I put her in the clothes dryer, and I shut the door. At least I didn't turn it on, thank God. So, I had my fun. I got back at her. But she was the "favored" child growing up. It was evident and contributed to how I was feeling. Disciplinary actions seemed unfair. I always got in trouble and was grounded or whatever. Sam seemingly got away with everything. It definitely felt worse for me because I was not biological.

When my girlfriends would come over, my room in Boca was in the front of the house and strategically chosen so I could sneak in and out the window when I wanted to. My sister's room was in the back of the house, and it was kind of scary back there. The house was on a canal, with no lights in the backyard and lots of bushes and trees. To a little kid, it would be pretty spooky. So, my friends and I would come around the house and bang really hard on her window and run away, so she thought ghosts, or something, were trying to get into her room. It was fun. In the long run, love wins the day. We got through all the crazy stuff that people do as kids, and now we are as close as sisters can be. I wouldn't trade her for anything.

I realized, some years ago, that Sam felt abandoned by me when I moved out. I didn't see it then because I was so caught up in my own shit, my own feelings. I didn't realize how it would have affected her. We've spoken about it. I think she understands now. It was never about her. Never would I have wanted to hurt her. She was very mad, hurt, and upset, but never said anything at the time. She doesn't talk about things. That is the one thing I wish she would do. I understand that she may not want to because she does not want to deal with the pain. It hurts. One of the reasons we bury it. I can definitely relate. My concern with her doing that is that she is sacrificing her own self-worth. Like Mom, she genuinely does not see what a remarkable woman she is.

So, while she lucked out with not having to deal with "T", she still did have her own issues with abandonment and love. Truth is, my sister was never without love, and she definitely was the spoiled kid, but not having the love of your biological father and having a good father, then losing him, is a lot to carry around. She and Mom fought too. It took me a lot of years and some real growing up to understand that I was not the only one who felt abandoned. There was plenty of abandonment feelings there to go around. I didn't want my sister ever to think that she wasn't loved because that's so far from the truth. She and I are Mom's whole heart.

Sam has given me a niece and a nephew, and they're the cutest things. I absolutely adore them. Arlene, "Lena", is seven, and Owen is two. Owen is the first boy in the family in 62 years, since my uncle Michael was born. All the other males married in. Even the pets are all girls. Lena is named after Grandma Arlene. The "L" in Lena is for Grandpa Larry. For as long as I can remember, Sam wanted to be a mom. At such a young age, I feel that she couldn't wait to be a mother. Much of why I feel this way is because of her feelings towards abandonment. She always said that she did not want to make the same mistakes that Mom did. While I'm sure that is true, every parent will make mistakes. I think sometimes because of the infighting at home and how she felt, a lack of discipline when needed may also contribute. Not disciplining and allowing no consequence will also produce their own set of problems. Mom did that with Sam because she did not want to be like Grandma Arlene. It becomes a never-ending cycle. Some actions have consequences, and they should. For example, time out or being grounded is appropriate when indicated. It does not mean you are a bad parent because you do so. It is quite the opposite. They will learn accountability. I hope Sam knows how wonderful a mother she is. Parenting is not easy by any means. It challenges you on all sorts of levels and in some cases makes you face your own skeletons. She is such an *amazing* mom, sister, and daughter.

We often carry around burdens that are not ours, but we think they are because of how they make us feel. Mom and Sam have theirs. Despite the years we were separated, Mom, Sam, and I are always there for each other, no matter what. Ironically, I diagnosed my sister's multiple sclerosis when she was 19. She called me up one day and was like, "Nikki, I can't see well out of one of my eyes." She had been drawing a lot more, and she thought maybe the eye trouble was related to that. I said, "Sam, you need to go see a doctor or to the hospital right now. You need to get this taken care of. This could be serious, possibly multiple sclerosis (MS)." I felt this way because of how she was describing her symptoms. I was still a student in school studying to become a PA. It turned out to be right. I am so thankful she was diagnosed early, and her MS is currently in remission. THANK GOD.

I couldn't imagine my life without Mom and Sam. They are such incredible women, and I am so proud of the women they have become. Afterall, I raised them :) That is the running joke in the family. Truth is, we raised each other. We complete and complement each other. For my mom, I love you so much. I wish for you to see the beautiful woman you are. While she still carries guilt of past mistakes, I am thankful for them. They led her to me. I would not know where I would be without her. Everything she has experienced in life has allowed her to take care of me and my sister, given her a heart that is so big, and has allowed her to relate to her patients. I hold no animosity, grudge, or resentment. Each of us does the best we can with what we know and what we have. Even during the challenging times, my sister and I were always in the forefront of her mind. She has sacrificed so much to make sure we had everything we needed. Growing up, yes, emotional maturity and understanding was lacking, however, she acted from what she was taught and how she felt about her place in life at that time. This has nothing to do with Sam or me. I am so proud of who she is.

I see her. All of her. Her strength, love, compassion, and resilience are admirable. She is my hero. My soulmate. I would change nothing about her. Each part of her life adds to the beautiful woman she is and has become. Much of my strength comes from her. Seeing her rebuild a life she loves and finally becoming happy is all I ever want from her. No more sacrifices. She's done that. I want her to live for her, to look in the mirror and see a woman who is a role model for others. She gave me a second chance at life.

Samantha is still in her growing phase. I am so proud of her. She has come so far and been through her own darkness. What I wish for her is for her to make peace with it. True peace. I want her to look in the mirror and see the strong, compassionate, loving, funny, talented woman I do. It is my hope for her that she will come to the realization in her own time that the things that happen to us are not what defines us. Mistakes are a part of life. Having a certain plan and coming to find out that the universe/God had others is part of the fun. This world needs more people with the heart she has. My sister is one that I admire. She too has not had an easy path and has her own darkness that she has faced coupled with her MS diagnosis. She is a fantastic mother to my niece and nephew, and I want her to show them how beautiful and resilient she is. No matter what happens to us in this life, we always have choices. Even if they are difficult ones. Time is something we don't have. We need to live our lives to the fullest. Take chances, step out of our comfort zone, and swap perspectives.

I love her more than she will ever know. Sam is my best friend, and I admire her. She has such a beautiful heart despite her past. It is time for her to heal too. She is seen. Valued. Loved. All parts of her. Stars only shine in the dark. I love her more than words could ever express and she, like Mom, completes me. I am so lucky to have her as a sister. In my weak moments, I kept Sam in the forefront of my mind. I wanted to be the kind of sister she deserved. So, everything I went through, I *had* to make it through. There was no other way. I had to persevere. I had to become someone Sam could be proud of, and plus, I had to keep raising her and Mom.

CHAPTER 12

RISING FROM THE PAIN
OF THE PANDEMIC

Being in Florida during the Pandemic was pretty awful. I experienced a lot of turmoil during those couple of years of never before experienced insanity that we all went through. I can speak for myself and probably the vast majority of my colleagues across the globe that the COVID-19 pandemic was terrible and traumatic. Honestly, my feelings and thoughts on medicine as a whole, after going through that, changed quite a bit. The trauma of what we saw during that awful time is the reason that a large part of healthcare providers left medicine. The general public will never truly understand what we on the front line did and how that has affected all of us in one way or another. Regardless of whether you're a nurse, a physician, a PA, a nurse practitioner, or respiratory therapist, it doesn't matter. We dedicate years, decades, of our lives to help others, to save them, giving our patients the best chance for quality of life. We know we are not God, and we can't control all the pieces, but we are supposed to make people better, and when you give everything that you have been taught to help a person, and it still doesn't work, repeatedly, it is probably one of the most defeating feelings ever. Doing what all of us healthcare providers do is not easy by any means. It is not just the education and time, but the emotional side of it as well. It is incredibly difficult not to let the bad days affect you. Every healthcare provider, regardless of profession type, has to keep moving through the day, no matter what happens. Imagine treating a critically ill patient, and God decides it is their time, providers carry the weight of that loss and have to move on and see the next patient. Each patient we have is deserving of our full attention. There is little time to process before the next patient. Imagine if there was a patient who came for one thing, and the universe took you by surprise, and the patient became critical. All of us who treat patients will always go over the events to be sure we did all the things to save them.

The life of a medical provider is incredibly emotionally taxing, normally. We all got into medicine to make a difference in some way, shape, or form. It doesn't matter if you are doing outpatient clinic, or surgery, dermatology, emergency medicine, critical care, we all chose this profession because we want to make a positive impact on the lives of others. We sacrifice ours for theirs. Thankfully, a good majority of the time we obtain outcomes we hoped for. The patient recovers to baseline or better, and they, their friends, and family can move forward with their lives.

Pre-pandemic, much of society respected healthcare providers and medicine and trusted what we said, did, etc. The pandemic changed a lot of that, unfortunately. I am not going to point fingers or blame anyone because that will not solve anything. But what I can tell you firsthand is that we *all* went through something that was unprecedented in modern times, and we did the best we could with something no one has ever faced before. Part of the doubt that has been instilled in the minds of many has to do with the ever-changing information. Things—everything—were changing faster than could be reported, and that unfortunately created so much confusion among the public, understandably. It was not medicine pulling the wool over anyone's eyes. You, society, were watching the evolution of a virus in real time. Every virus does it. Some are faster than others. Medicine typically studies them and adjusts as information arises or changes. Think of a common virus like the Influenza virus. Most common variations from the prior year help to create the vaccine by trying to predict, with pretty great odds most years, what the new possible combination of genes will be, so we can keep society safe. Most of the time, the vaccine for the flu is very effective. Vaccination does not mean you won't get the disease. Nothing in medicine is 100%. Some protection is much better than none at all, and if symptoms do arise, they are usually very mild and short-lived. Can people develop a reaction? Yes. But that is true for anything. You can eat a banana and have an allergic reaction. People will argue they don't want to put "chemicals" in their body, but *everything* is a chemical. Acetaminophen, sugar substitutes, carbohydrates, very familiar things... yet, not considered dangerous because of their familiarity. Truth be told, many common medications over the counter are dangerous when used improperly. So, placing an "unfair" label on something that *saves* lives is, in my humble opinion, a mistake and dangerous.

The other thing to consider is the value assigned to familiar viruses. Society takes these things for granted. Because many alive now have not seen what these viruses are capable of, due to vaccination. Measles is deadly. Mumps causes sterility in males, among other things. The influenza virus is dangerous. It kills people, too. Thousands. But it is not common to associate death/danger with the flu because of vaccines and familiarity. The Mono virus is another common and very dangerous one. Unless someone has known a person who suffered complications like heart failure, death from it, it is too underestimated. The Epstein-Barr virus that causes mono has also been a potential link to some autoimmune disorders, like multiple sclerosis, in addition to being suspected to be a cause of a whole host of diseases.

In the situation with the pandemic, this was an entirely new "animal" we were dealing with. We needed to see what the heck it was, how it was contracted, then make small groups of certain criteria to look for patterns, prevalence in age groups, certain countries, isolating where it originated from. Further, needing to decode it to see what it is, is there a close family of viruses we can compare to and so much more. These things take time. Days, weeks for results.

Think if you've ever been to a specialist and they order a gambit of labs for one reason or another. They take time to see results. That is the limitation of technology. This thing spread faster than we could retrieve information, and by the time that information came out, there was already new information we needed to process. So, you take that delay, coupled with fear and you have a recipe for disaster. This was never before seen. I really do not think society, most outside of medicine, truly grasps that. Even still, we healthcare providers went to work every day not knowing if we would return, or possibly bring this thing home and transmit it to loved ones, all to save your lives. I personally worked three weeks straight, 12-hour shifts, many times longer and driving an hour each way to and from work. More often than not, days run about 14 or 16hours. We do not leave when the clock reveals a time. I was sleeping at hotels because I did not want to infect anyone in my family. My nickname during the pandemic was Nic-Covid because I worked so many shifts right in the middle of these sick patients. I am not sure if I ever had the virus. If I did, I did not have any symptoms. I knew what I signed up for. I knew the risks. So did many of us. Did we ever think we would actually encounter something of this magnitude in our lifetime with modern day medicine? Nope. We all were scared. We did not know if we would return home, and many didn't.

I was doing emergency medicine at that time, and I was seeing patients in the ER and parking lot before we had the tent with these patients, depending how it was scheduled. I put myself out there more often than not, because I was not letting my pregnant colleagues out there, and those with children, increasing chances for exposure. We were short providers who became sick right off the bat, and I was covering physician and PA shifts.

At that time, it was in the very early stages of testing for the virus, working with our infectious disease team and CDC to test so that we could obtain the most accurate information. You cannot just go and screen everyone. You will never have correct data. You need to minimize variables at first, receive information, and expand as you know more. For those that did not qualify, I was cursed at, spit on, called all sorts of horrific names, and had chairs thrown at me. I did not take it personally at first, but eventually it does make you feel awful. Some lied about being infected and spit on staff. Humanity showed both of its sides during the pandemic. Much of these reactions from people were out of fear. With that said, it in no way excuses their behavior. All over the world, colleagues on the front line experienced much of the same. We were not only trying to decode this thing but trying to figure out how to treat it too. From the beginning, we, medicine, were at a disadvantage. We saw a lack of everything, information, supplies, staff because they were getting sick, many very ill and many died too all across the globe. Then, you have the "regular" patients too in addition to patients who were fearful to come in and be seen because they did not want to catch this thing. It was a disaster from every single angle. Administrators tried. Medicine tried. We gave *everything* for the world. We gave all of ourselves, even a piece of our hearts.

I think one of the worst things providers experienced was not just what I mentioned above, but now the hospitals were full, everything was scarce, and people were dying. Outside a pandemic, in normal life, it's awful to lose a patient. But here we were, where no family was able to see their loved ones or be with them during their final moments in many cases. No one should ever have to experience that. Alone, with a lack of human connection, it broke our hearts. We stayed with our patients at their bedside and, in many cases, were able to use iPads and iPhones to video call with patients' families. We had to minimize spread, and we were heartbroken for them to not have our patient's family at their bedside.

Everyone suffered. Healthcare professionals carry the weight of all of that on our hearts. Family members passed, colleagues passed, our police, PAs, firefighters, nurses, paramedics, physicians, and patients were dying or becoming gravely ill, despite giving all we have been trained to do to help them, because this virus was novel, never before seen. We, in medicine, had to learn as we went. Medical providers across the globe were sharing what worked and what did not for our patients. All of us were struggling. Imagine doing all you can, working as hard as we were, but it still was not good enough. But you have to keep going. There is no time to process those things. All that mattered was their lives. There were so many patients who needed us. Our feelings were pushed down and compartmentalized because we had to stay focused. We had to be strong for them.

I almost became a patient a few times because of low blood sugar and dehydration. Taking off the PPE and putting it back on was a chore, and that too was scarce across the globe, patients needed us. *Lunch? Water? Bathroom breaks? What is that?* Time was not our friend. This virus initially seemingly preferred certain ages and some with certain medical histories. But, even then, it changed. It evolved and then "chose" to have a predilection for pregnant women, pediatrics, and young adults. It went after everyone at some point. Take all of that physical and emotional stress and couple or triple it with being hit, kicked, spit on, sprayed with antiseptics, and then conspiracy theories of how it was not real or it was a hoax. That would make you feel defeated, wanting to give up. We were running on fumes to try to reunite families safely. Medicine is traumatized from it, that I promise. Some more than others. Each are dealing with it in different ways. The false and delayed information created a divide between society and medicine. It is terrible.

Unfortunately, the consequences of this pandemic will span generations. Why? It will take a long time to re instill "faith" in us and to see the actual results of things less spoken about like the younger generations not having social interactions for so long, suicides, financial constraints, and so much more. It will take a long time to really see the long-term effects. We did everything we could do with information, technology, supplies, and staff we had. We fought. Until we couldn't.

Multiple times, I thought I was going to catch it. I remember when my mask got ripped off one day, and shortly after, I sent my family a text of my wishes if I caught the virus or died from it. I am so glad that we are "over" the pandemic, despite its effects still lingering in society. Fear makes people do crazy things. Yet, we are five almost six years later and the divide is still present. It is my opinion that our lifelines during that time were the ones who sent food, drinks, even the simple thank you. All forms of gratitude and appreciation, those simple acts, meant more to us than anyone will ever know. It kept us going. Overall, I am incredibly proud of medicine as a whole. Despite everything, we kept going. We kept fighting for our patients, our loved ones, and our colleagues. We had to succeed. There was no other choice. To all my colleagues around the world, I see you and am so very thankful for all you do.

Despite knowing the risks of having a career in medicine, I knew exactly what I was getting myself into, but it weighs on you. I understand why healthcare providers have left medicine. I worry for the future of healthcare overall. We are scarce, funding is being cut, and there is a severe physician shortage—especially in infectious disease, emergency medicine, and primary care. Infectious disease had so many vacancies for match this year. If we have another pandemic, which I'm sad to say is very likely, we are in trouble. Worldwide. I don't think we are prepared, especially in the current climate. Sorry, whatever you believe, I am not making this political but what is happening is setting us up for big trouble. Politicizing medicine was and is a large problem contributing to the overall problem then and now. One thing only is true regarding that is *politics has no place in medicine.* Politics **should not** make medical decisions. Cutting funding, limiting access to education, research... We as a society will feel it for decades. Discussing healthcare is not politics, regardless of topic. That is another dangerous situation the pandemic created. Combining the two puts' lives at risk. Period. Medicine is not the "enemy."

Food for thought, it is not only physically and mentally taxing to be in medicine, but also expensive for providers and the patients. In a post-pandemic world, everything costs more. People having to choose paying their rent or paying for medication/healthcare should not even be a topic for discussion. I am a registered independent. Not a fan of either side to be honest, both have played their parts in the current situation we find ourselves in. Political parties need revamping. With that said, Americans should never have to be in a position where they have to choose their livelihood or health. I am not sure if there is one correct answer for the issues that we all find ourselves in, but what I do know is that we have to do it *united*. The pandemic is also, in my humble opinion, responsible for the worsening individualistic mindset that affects so many these days, an underestimated adverse effect arising from it. Everyone is stressed out. The thing is, we are all worried about the same things yet feel that no one understands. We are all in this together, and what we do affects others' lives, directly or indirectly, whether we realize that or not. Together is the *only* way through this.

CHAPTER 13

PASSION FROM THE EMBERS, FORGING PURPOSE IN THE FIRE

EMERGING FROM THE ASHES

I was minding my own business when the universe decided to plant another seed, opening the door to earning the doctorate. I met this man who planted the initial idea which was completely unexpected. While I knew that the PA-Doctorate existed, at the time, I was content, happy with my position, my team, and things were comfortable. Well, the universe had other ideas and deposited that seed through a man who I met through some atypical circumstances. While I am not ethically allowed to give details, our conversation began with, "You have the same eyes. She keeps saying you two have the same eyes." Now there were only two people in the world who knew the significance of that phrase: Mom and Grandma Arlene. "You have the same eyes," he kept repeating. I was in shock. Speechless for probably one of the first times in my life. I could not figure it out. *How does this man know private details about me?* These are things that were not known outside my family, not on the internet, or anywhere. He began to tell me more. It was as if he had *been* a part of my whole life up to that point. Now, I am not a stranger to odd phenomena like this, but never did I ever think that *this*, let alone the location and timing of what was happening, would occur. I was silent. I did not ask questions. He spoke. I listened.

Thank goodness I had a witness because otherwise, no one would've believed me. In the middle of it, he mentioned he was a medium. I was floored. It made sense. He turned to the witness I had with me and told her, "Stop fighting with your fiancé. You two are going to get married, and you will figure out a place to live." She teared up. She looked at me in disbelief. Shocked. Apparently, she and her fiancé had an argument that was coming up frequently that month about just that. She was hoping he would propose, and they could not settle on where they would live. We looked at each other, both with tears in our eyes, in awe. He continued to tell me that I was going to earn my doctorate and that I was going to write this book. Neither of these things were on my radar. The idea of the book and doctoral degree was not anything I had considered before this interaction. This man knew intimate details of my life. My biological donor, biological father, the bullying, and even that my sister (who had no idea at the time) was pregnant with my nephew. This was significant because she was just a few weeks along at the time. Hearing these things, what are the odds of this being a coincidence?

Exactly one week later, another unusual meeting occurred. A woman, who was just incredible for so many reasons, also oddly exclaimed that I was going to "become a doctor." This woman was amazing. She grew up in a time when women were not allowed to do much of anything. They were able to become doctors but were limited in their specialty. She and I spoke about her life, and I was in awe. She told me that she wanted to be a surgeon, but at that time, women were only allowed to become pediatricians or OBGYNs. She rolled her eyes at that and told me that she "gave in to the societal norms," entered into marriage, had "the kids", and was a homemaker. She loved being a wife and mother. However, she said that she always felt like something was missing. Some years after the birth of her son, she went back to school and earned her bachelor's. When her son was older, she and her then-husband divorced, and she went back to school and earned two PhDs. The divorce was mutual, she exclaimed, "We drifted apart, and when my son left the house, it was evident." One of her PhDs was in engineering and the other in astrophysics. I was shocked and in awe of her. I love meeting strong women. Through every culture across time and the globe, the one group of people that have always been restricted are women, and here was this remarkable woman who took advantage of things that became available to her, building a legacy and paving the way for other women in a time of lack for women. She went on to tell me that, ultimately, she worked for NASA and helped to design one of the first circuit boards. Wow! What an amazing woman. I love women who do things like that against the odds, who just go against the grain and shatter those glass ceilings, because that's what it needs to be. We don't honor intellect and critical thinking in general in this country. Society doesn't like smart people, and more often than not, we negate the intelligence of women. It's really sad. Through all of time, across cultures and the globe, women have always been scrutinized and seen as inferior. So, when I meet strong, empowering women, it lights my world up. We are too hard on ourselves, too critical of others, and we should be lifting each other, sharing our stories, and celebrating women. Lifting another woman up does not take away from us. It adds value, to her, to you, and to everyone she empowers. Afterall, we are remarkable. No one can light up a room the way a woman does when she walks in. Especially one that is empowered.

I related to her. I respected her. Despite the differences, the underlying theme remains the same: a woman trying to defy the odds and become a ripple in the pond. Randomly, she told me I was going to get my doctorate. I chuckled and told her I was content where I was. She smiled and said, "You'll see; you're going to go back." I couldn't help but think that the universe was planting another seed with signs to get me to move. *What was I being prepared for?*

Whelp, she was right. He was, too. Believe me, I tried to fight it. The two and their words circled and circled in my head. So, I gave in to the universe and signed up for the professional pathway at ATSU. Time flew. I loved my classes. In the last two years, my professional growth has been amazing. I found a love for education and quality improvement, and became a published PA. Graduating and walking across that stage was surreal. Never did I ever think that would happen. I still have to look at my diploma.

The purpose of my doctorate was to help others in every way I could, based on my life experiences and education. I earned my GED after being jumped and feeling afraid to return to school, despite attending night school. I tried college twice but dropped out again because I was intimidated and didn't think I was good enough, especially after Ryan said to me, "Oh, look, the high school dropout is back!" That was one of the most intimidating moments. I was already insecure about everything academic, and when I enrolled at university, I faced this guy who, by the way, knew nothing about *why* I dropped out. Being jumped and dealing with PTSD made walking through high school halls to attend classes, even at night, extremely difficult. The walls felt like they were closing in, I couldn't breathe, my face tingled, my heart raced, and I thought I might pass out. When I finally thought I had gathered the courage to try college again, that man's comment made me apprehensive all over again.

ETERNAL HOPE, TRANSFORMATION, AND RESILIENCE

Over the years, there have been so many challenges, tests, heartbreaks, and disappointments that genuinely made me feel and think all sorts of things. Ranging from *"Why me? Not again! OK, Let's do this, perhaps I am not meant to do this. Maybe I am not good enough, smart enough,"* and each time, I pushed through it. There were so many times when I wanted to give up on life too. I am very honest about that. I struggled a lot. My emotions were all over the place for years. I had such a difficult time trying to make sense of things. I could not understand why I had to experience all of these things to the degree they were from such a young age. It never really made sense, yet, regardless, I kept going. I held on to hope and knew things had to improve at some point. When I was accepted into PA school, I cannot even begin to say how happy I was. I felt a sense of accomplishment. The journey was not without trials and tribulations, but in my mind, finally, I was here. Life was getting started. The harder things got, the better I did.

Finally, the tough times were over. I completed school, graduated with academic honors, and won so many other awards at graduation. PA school did not come with the same drama that ultrasound did. I was hired in 2016 as an ER PA at a hospital system that is world-renowned. To me, life was getting better. *Smooth sailing,* I thought. Shortly after being hired, there were some major changes within my department, and I had to step it up. For a year, I worked around 21 twelve-hour shifts a month. Our patients needed us, short-staffed for a little while, a colleague was out on maternity, and another was moving because her husband got into a residency program in another state. It was tough eight months out of school, and honestly, I am thankful for it. As scary as it was, I think it made me a stronger provider. Things began to settle some and the new hires were starting. There were a lot of positive changes. A few months later, in 2018, Dad got sick out of nowhere. I was also asked to help in another department because one of their providers was going to be on maternity. I said yes. I was nervous and would be working (because I chose it) full time for both departments. For three months, I did it. Furthermore, I was in the American Academy of PAs House of Delegates as a delegate and alternate, as well as on the board of directors for the Florida Academy of PAs as south regional director, eventually becoming the vice president. My team and I did all kinds of community events. Now, Dad was sick. I was still doing all those things, and more, when that happened. He was admitted to a local hospital for a urinary infection. I found that weird because, for the most part, healthy men do not usually get them. While I was caring for him in the hospital and doing the other things I mentioned, I was stressed. I was not eating much and just trying to go through the motions. I just wanted Dad home. Healthy. Around this time, while I felt like the universe just kept handing me boulders to hold, a colleague filed a false and exaggerated report on me. I know who she is, and even though she did what she did, I forgive her. Why? Because doing that to a "friend" tells more about her struggles and insecurities. It is not about me. She does not like her reflection when she sees me. I just walk away because I know karma will come around. In the meantime, continuing to be a catalyst for positive change. I took a little bit of processing to see, and when it was happening, I was feeling all sorts of things. I cannot speak to all the details, but I can tell you, thankfully, everything worked out. But, *what in the world…?* I thought. Here, in my mind, I was trying to help the departments, Dad was sick with another hospital mismanaging his care, and this? *What was the lesson?* I thought. Dad passed away during that time. I took a little time off work and returned. 2019 was awful too. What I knew I wanted was to be sure to take care of myself this time when grieving. I didn't with Grandpa, and I wanted to be sure to learn from my past mistakes. I thought I handled it. I definitely did better than before. I admit to pushing some people away, but not as severely as previously. I spoke up more. But I admit that I did bury myself in work. The way I saw it then was that I was still "new" and needed to "prove myself." I didn't realize I was actually hiding. Most of 2019 was dealing with Dad's estate and trying to be patient with myself. Then, 2020 came. The Pandemic. For a large part of it I was in the ER, but then our surgical ICU (SICU) needed help. I was asked to go. Scared, I went. For a while I was doing ER and SICU. Plus still trying to grieve. There wasn't time for that, though. Everyone needed us. So, I kept going.

After being there for some time, I noticed some changes in one of the team members. Not that it would be something that I would necessarily get involved in. But it was starting to affect work. I brought up a concern that she may be going through something, and I was worried about her to a senior member of the team, and unfortunately, he used it as an opportunity to behave poorly. To make a long story short and to limit details I am unable to share, this senior, who we will call "N", was not behaving in a way a person of that status should. It was awful for weeks. For the first time in a very long time, I questioned my sanity. In my mind, I am here to help. Concerns were brought it up and it was not received in the way I thought it would be. I was not eating well, hardly sleeping because of the actions of this person. One night, I felt flushed, my heart was racing, and I couldn't breathe. I went outside, tried to catch a breath, and literally screamed to the universe, "Dad, Grandpa, whatever the heck this is for, it better show itself!" My Apple Watch tracked my heart in the 190s. I was really struggling with trying to find the positive. If anyone heard me, they would have committed me. That was the last boulder. I felt like I was falling. I couldn't get up. I couldn't hold anymore. I really thought I was going to give up this time. So much came all at once, and truth be told, I did not provoke any of it. The problem was that I was trying to be everything to everyone, and it was not reciprocated. In my professional or personal life, the problem with being the strong one is that no one checks on you. Because it seems you always have it handled. But this was my breaking point. Or it was the beginning of a new transformation. Literally, the very next day, an amazing opportunity arose, and I took it. That brought me to internal medicine. I was excited. It was as if the universe responded to that plea for help. As far as the senior colleague goes, karma said hello.

I love my position on the hospitalist team. I was able to help throughout on the observation unit, utilizing my experiences in the prior departments to help facilitate positive change. There have been some small hurdles, but nothing like what I previously experienced until recently.

Because I am writing this after it has all completed, but still with missing information, there may be some gaps. But essentially, another (or perhaps the same one) anonymous colleague filed another report. I cannot get into the details, but what I can say is that it was fabricated, unfounded, and all from hearsay and gossip. I am not sure what set this person off. I know who it is. I am not surprised, but am, in the same breath, if that makes sense. This person is a gossip and has been known to put down others on social media. I had to stop it when they tried to spread some rumors about another colleague. Honestly, that could be what happened. This person has issues with professionalism and just runs her mouth. Anyone to fabricate lies to try to "take down" a "friend" in the manner she did is not a good person. At all. God saw it, and she will have to answer to him. Meanwhile, I will continue to move forward and continue to be a light in the lives of others.

I have been on both sides of gossip and it's an awful place to be. So, this person has a history of these things and these days it does not take much for people to be cruel. Thankfully, the investigation found nothing. As for that person, I will pray for them and keep leveling up. I don't do revenge or anger, or any of those other things. Why? Why would I? What is the reason? It doesn't make anything better, and it gives our power away. I don't and won't stoop to that level. I have worked so hard to be where I am, and I refuse to give my power away to low-vibrational individuals. That is what they want. My response? Silence and keep paying it forward. Keep mentoring and being a positive light for others. There is no need to be like them. Offering forgiveness and praying that they find happiness is best. Because people who do those things, in my humble opinion, are unhappy. They try to bring others down. Some are jealous. Those feelings are between them and their God. There is enough room at the top for us all. I will continue to support women and not be a "mean girl."

Over the years, I have become a leader in many ways. Interestingly, that was never my plan. I wanted to know who I was, searching for a sense of self, searching for love. Through all the adversities, I chose to overcome them. The result was becoming a leader in the community. So, what kind of a leader would I be if I behaved like those lower vibrational people? Not a very good one. To me, leadership shows others the way, building up those who need, fostering growth and positive changes, planting the seeds to be cultivated for tomorrow. Going through all I have over my lifetime so far has prepared me for this. Leading others, becoming an empath with a strong intuition, helping others heal, that is my purpose. I will continue to let others know they are not alone in the dark. I will continue to be the lighthouse.

Each of us comes into this life with possibilities. A sense of purpose. Love. An unbridled desire to explore possibilities. Life, it happens. Circumstances arise that are meant to challenge us, allow us to grow or falter to the difficulty that lies before us. Looking at your reflection and seeing someone who once was, choosing a variety of courses that is thought to be correct based on the limited and biased information in front of us, is where failure, doubts, and weaknesses thrive. But holding still long enough allows us to see a glimmer of light in the dark. Yin is not without yang; summer is not without winter. Everything must change to grow, and it is the perspective that we choose to find the beauty in the storm. The energy, the force of change it produces, if you allow, will yield purpose. That view is unmatched. Embracing challenges and facing every moment that lies in front of you with clarity, even when it's cloudy, is important. Trust in yourself, in God, the universe, a divine plan that is far beyond ego. Written in the stars, destiny is revealed. Utilizing all that has been learned so others can feel safe, comforted, and know they are not alone on their journey as it unfolds, and they step into their power despite the odds, is invigorating and brings you back to a sense of purpose that you entered this life for.

It is worth it. Every time. No one should be ashamed of who they are. The challenges and choices made are not to be ashamed of. Because you have found your beauty, your purpose through the pain. You are the phoenix.

Purpose

124

CHAPTER 14

BUILT FROM THE EMBERS OF PAIN, IGNITED BY POWER

I graduated from A. T. Still University (ATSU) in August of 2024 with my doctorate as a PA. After earning my doctorate, not much changed clinically. I'm still doing all the things I was doing before. I see my patients, diagnose, treat, and prescribe medications. If anything has changed, it's my perspective within the organization. I find that now, I can be of greater impact. Having earned my Doctor of Medical Science degree opens a lot of doors within the organization and outside it. While I am not sure where this new path will lead, having this degree will allow me to make the greatest impact in helping others. To me, that is my "why"… utilizing my personal and professional experiences to make a positive difference in another's life. Being the catalyst, the ripple in the pond, positively impacting the lives of others, leaves my imprint on the world.

Earning the PA doctorate, in conjunction with my prior clinical and life experiences, has enabled me to undertake and implement larger projects than I would have been able to accomplish previously. Not because it was restricted, but due to a lack of perspective and confidence. Having worked in six specialties as a PA and my time as a sonographer provided a unique perspective, which I didn't know at the time, would yield these ideas that will benefit our patients, staff, and the organization. I am thankful to work for an enterprise that values PAs, supports professional growth, and encourages us to work to the top of our license. Earning my doctorate is something I never thought I would achieve. Never did I ever think I was capable.

However, the universe had a different plan...

Looking back, I believe it was either a test from the universe or a redirection. Perhaps "life" needed to happen first because while I felt ready, I really wasn't. Honestly, if I had kept attending classes going straight through, I probably would have failed out. The catastrophe that would have followed could have deterred me or potentially changed my path entirely.

You see, what I have learned is that delays, while they can be frustrating, sad, and heartbreaking, oftentimes, there is a silver lining. There is something you need to learn, do, prepare, and strengthen before the next phase can occur. So, even though I was annoyed and intimidated by Ryan's comment back then, looking back, I'm thankful. Years later, I returned to school and earned my associate's degree as a Diagnostic Medical Sonographer, followed by board certifications in multiple specialties and becoming one of the best in my field, eventually deciding to continue my studies, setting my sights on becoming a PA after about nine years as a sonographer.

I graduated summa cum laude from Barry University's undergraduate program with multiple academic honors and was finally accepted into Barry's PA program, also graduating with my master's in science with academic honors and won multiple awards for academics and philanthropic work I had done.

Applying to PA school was its own challenge. Several situations could have easily made me give up. I was even told by a local university's PA admissions counselor that she "found it hard to believe" when I mentioned my GPA. I had called to inquire about criteria not listed on their site, and when she asked my GPA—which was a 3.7 overall at the time—that was her response. After hearing that, I officially withdrew my application and screenshot my unofficial transcript showing my GPA. Maybe it was a bold move, but to me, who was she to say that? Removing my application was because I wanted a program that would help me build a strong foundation to then help others. Her comment was honestly upsetting, and I didn't want to be part of a university that had someone like that working there, especially in admissions. The face of the university should be someone uplifting, encouraging, and honest. Not the Negative Nelly she was. During the interview phase of the application process, I was asked to visit one of the elite programs in the Northeast. I was so excited, and it was my first one. I was the second to last interview, and I remember walking into the office with two other professors on the admissions team. I was elated. Nervous, but the good kind. I earned my place here. All the hard work, dedication, and personal growth led me here. I was on cloud nine. However, that excitement was short lived. One of the interviewers asked me to explain "the discrepancy with my high school grades." I was confused. I remember thinking, *does he have the right application?* Well, I asked him exactly that. This interview was nothing of what I would have expected.

Sure, I figured they would ask about my GED, dropping out of high school, etc. I never thought I would hear what came next. When I asked the professor what he meant, I clarified and informed him that I did not complete high school, and he must have the wrong application information. He then asked, " Why didn't you complete it?" Well, there it was, the can of worms I opened. *Why couldn't I just keep my mouth shut?* I thought. I briefly gave a rundown of some of the obstacles I had overcome that were pertinent to the question and the program. I stayed strong. Positive. But he was not having it. He continued to probe more and more. Here, I thought I would be discussing the straight As for the last four years, all the community things I was involved in, leadership, everything. Contrast that with my past; it is quite the journey; one I am proud of. But instead, his next question was, "I see you are thirty something and have no kids yet, how do you feel about that?" Ok, wait a second, *what?!* I kind of see what he was doing, here is a rigorous program, with an extensive amount of time that would be needed, and perhaps he wanted to see if I was interested in having kids, where my priorities were, or perhaps because my grades were so great, he was picking at anything to try to get inside my head and see how I would react. It was intimidating. Infuriating. I had done all this hard work, overcame all these things, and this is what he was focused on? Not the genetics and epigenetics research I've done, my grades, mentoring, leadership things, how I got to that point. No. He wanted to see why a thirty-something "old" woman was applying to PA school instead of having children. Perhaps that was not his intention. But that is how it felt. I was so frustrated that I began to tear up. I truly felt unseen. All of the positive I had done, and quite honestly, I was not really sure what I was expecting, but not that. I couldn't wait for the interview to be over. Slowly but surely, I built my confidence, refusing to let someone else decide *my* future. I was accepted into the program. I respectfully declined. That was not a place where I would become my best self. Instead of feeling intimidated, I used it as motivation. Just like I did with the Keiser dean. I was accepted to my first choice as well, Barry University. I could not wait to begin. I enjoyed my undergraduate stay, and the professors truly invest in the students. They are challenging, but in a good way. They support you through all the things needed to strengthen the foundation when becoming your best version. Now, here I was, graduating from ATSU with my doctorate. I couldn't believe it. **From GED to doctorate—what an achievement**. My younger self is proud.

THE WELLNESS GARDEN PROJECT

The doctorate has enabled me to work on several projects at the hospital that I am very proud of. One is a community therapeutic and wellness garden for the patients, staff, students, community, and anyone else who needs a place to decompress. I love gardening. It's one of my favorite hobbies, and my happy place. Perhaps I was a fairy or something in some prior life. The idea came about on a random day. My office overlooks one of the plazas on the hospital campus; it's beautiful. The date palms, the architecture, and the lighting, it really is a beautiful space. But it could use some love. My perspective in the different departments as a PA and previously in radiology contributed to the idea because it allowed me to see patients under different services and in a variety of acuity levels. Add the pandemic in addition to how all feel in this "new" society… Everyone is under pressure these days. Financial, social, you name it. Further, many of our patients are critical and here for weeks, sometimes months. Staff in any hospital always tries to boost morale of the patients when they are there, especially for that long. We try to brighten up their day how we can. But those white walls can make you feel institutionalized. Having a space to feel the sun, hear the birds, see waterscapes in the background, tropical plants such as bougainvillea, orchids on the trees, bromeliads, lush foliage, flowers for other pops of color and all the other beautiful and esthetically pleasing things.

Not to get "nerdy," but the literature supports these kinds of gardens. It improves overall health and well-being for everyone. These types of gardens have proven to improve mood, energy levels, patient experience, improve morbidity and mortality, and fosters a positive mindset, reduces the length of stay, allowing our patients and us to heal. Plus, this is an overall win for the institution. The garden's purpose is to provide a space that is calm, relaxing, and rejuvenating for both our patients and staff. While the hospital has serenity rooms, a chapel, and all that, it's not the same. Science proves that being outdoors is definitely better for improving the overall health and wellbeing of the individual. There is nothing like feeling the sun on your face after having been in a hospital for so long. The warmth is comforting, soothing, and provides a feeling of gratitude never previously felt. Anyone who has been hospitalized, or who knows someone who has for an extended period of time, understands this feeling of helplessness, this lack of independence. When they go outside for the first time, feeling the wind, the warmth of the sun, and hearing the birds... it is refreshing. You're free. It reenergizes you and melts away all the immediate stress, allowing the person to refocus, recharge, and realign with their healing journey.

THE ACUTE PAIN PROJECT

Another project that I have going is the acute pain project. This project has many parts. This also grew from the various perspectives as a PA in the hospital, in addition to my life experiences. When I teach my students, I'm very big on bias, especially within the medical field. We're all human with different upbringings, cultures, familiarities, training, and education. Therefore, how a patient is "seen" varies greatly across the board, and vice versa, how a patient "sees" the provider. So, what do I mean by this? Well, when we are training, we are taught that history is everything. This is true; however, I will argue it. History is only as good as the person asking the questions and as good as the one answering them. Just because a question is asked does not mean that the person answering will give the desired answer. Nor does it mean that the definition of the words chosen is the same as the person interpreting.

So, where does this leave the provider? Sounds a bit complicated, right? It is. The provider has to take everything in. Culture, age, physical exam, the history provided, and so much more. Additionally, the provider needs to learn to obtain the information to gather the story and put the pieces together. There is a lot that can affect the outcome. Another important factor is the onset of the disease, in particular. I never like to play "Monday morning quarterback" and assume anything. Perhaps the person(s) the patient saw before did what they thought was best based on the information they had. Often, diseases don't like to present what they really are... until they do.

Sadly, with how medicine is changing, the increased demand of patients, insurance companies, and the severe lack of everyone in the medical field, and specialization of medicine adds to the challenges. Each patient gets less time with their provider, and often this puts both the patient and the provider at a disadvantage. It's terrible, and believe it or not, it's not anything that's within a hospital's control. It's the insurance companies that are driving these things, and now politics. Bias has existed way before these changes and evolving medical environments and patient needs and is affected by literally everything.

So, why is this project so important? For example, if a patient comes in and let's say they have low back pain, the first thing that people are going to think of is muscular strain, sciatica pain, or something else in the musculoskeletal department. Well, the reality is it could be something fatal, like an aortic dissection, or another fatal disorder if misdiagnosed, called May-Thurner, which is a little less well-known. A cough, for example, could be endocarditis, an infection in the heart. "Dizziness" could be an abnormal rhythm in the heart or even a pulmonary embolus (blood clot in the lung). Aside from chief complaint bias, there is this unfortunate divide between the patient and provider to no intentional fault of either.

Overall, many medical providers often don't have a good idea and/ or are not comfortable when it comes to treating acute or chronic pain. The reason for that is that many, many moons ago, medicine as a whole created this unintentional divide when they tried to backtrack on the whole narcotics situation. When medicine as a whole decided to "fix" the situation, it inadvertently created an unintentional divide between the patient and provider, and both feel judged. The patient often when "pain" terminology is heard, the patient assumes the provider is thinking they are "seeking" and the guard immediately goes up. Also, there is an automatic assumption and relationship to "pain" and narcotics. However, there are a whole host of ways to treat acute pain. Medicine as a whole, in an effort not to create more addiction, there is a hesitance in prescribing controlled substances across the board, even continuing what a patient takes from home. Also, the underutilization of multi-modal analgesia (using multiple types of medications to treat pain), rarely used medications such as IV acetaminophen. Other, less familiar medications, such as those in the antipsychotic realm, are also not utilized much. Multiple factors contribute to this, such as the cost of medication, habit, and familiarity of the provider, not being on formulary, to name a few. You will see more of the utilization of opiate alternatives in the treatment of acute pain; however, despite the state and federal requirements, providers are still not really comfortable in doing so. This, coupled with chief complaint bias, adds to the problem.

This is what I am trying to bring to light. Providers and patients have the same goals. To feel better and to get our patients to feel better. We are all on the same team. Therefore, I want to continue to educate nurses, residents, PAs, nurse practitioners, and even physicians about how, what, when, and why should help the relationship between the patient and provider. Well, at least that is my hope. Once there is a recognition that unintentional bias exists, and all are guilty of it, patients and providers. The relationship will improve all around. Recognition, acceptance, and understanding of all things potentially involved that can affect will, over time, improve.

CHAPTER 15

EMBERS LIGHTING THE WAY

In addition to my day-to-day work, I teach and mentor. I love it. I work with students of all levels of education, from high school, college, and graduate and medical school. I mentor young men and women who are aspiring to be a PA, thinking about it, or even considering going to medical school or other healthcare career.

I've come to see that everything I've been through has allowed me to "see" certain things in people, strengthened my intuition, and led me to be a mentor the future of medicine. I remember what it was like, trying to figure out your place in the world and carrying around a whole host of insecurities, in some cases burdens that are not even theirs to carry just hoping to find the right path. I see now that it is my purpose to help, heal, and guide. It is interesting because each of my mentees and students has needed a push, advice, or motivation that I was able to provide. Not your typical student things. These were parts of them that they never said out loud. My past and the whole host of obstacles that at some times nearly veered me off my path gave me an insight, an intuition about things. I always tell my students that I will find their weakness and strengthen it. After all, their strengths don't need the attention. They will laugh and many times brush it off, but by the end of their rotations with me, their insecurities are strengthened, they are clinically stronger and confident in the fact that we are all a work in progress, and that is OK. More often than not, much of the insecurity's providers have is never wanting to miss anything, never wanting to harm the patient. That is largely in the forefront of most students. However, most of us in medicine are some variations of a type A. So why does that matter? Well, because we want to control, we want to fix everything. We got into this career to make others' lives better. Each of us wants to be the very best we can. But when you hold on so tightly, guided by fear, you will never grow to the full potential. Especially when fear is dictating every step. We need to let go a little. Understand that we are all human and make mistakes. Just as in life, things can happen, and people can get hurt. So, what I tell them is that when you truly accept that you are flawed, mistakes will be made but the likelihood of the chance of a mistake will significantly increase if you let the fear drive. But recognizing our flaws and weak points, strengthening them, realizing that we are all learning, and we are all feeling the same way, as you go through your training, you will be freed of fears' hold. Knowing, recognizing, and accepting mistakes happen, allowing fear to be a motivator rather will give you the best experiences during training and with your patients. Because you will not be afraid to jump in and learn. Many of us, when we are training, are nervous and unsure. We want to be seen in a good light. We do not want our mentors, professors, and preceptors to think we are not capable. Every student has that fear. Reality and perspective really are feelings we do to ourselves. That is the fear that is driving. Release it. The truth is, when we let go of what we think others think of us, and the fear of doing something wrong, we are free. Learning all that we can to truly be the best version of ourselves for our patients and the team we are on.

This is something that I learned through my training, but more through my life experiences. Everything has led me here. Being comfortable with your dark and light is something many of us need to do. We tend to shy away from healing or even accepting the flawed parts of us, but that is what makes us imperfectly perfect. Too often, we carry around the burdens of others placed upon us, and we assign ourselves a value from it. We need to stop that. By sharing with them and giving them the courage and strength to pursue this amazing career, understanding that the entire way we will be challenged, we will grow, we will make mistakes, and that is okay. Failure, and I know a lot about this topic because I did everything wrong first, is not a weakness. Not recognizing that it provides an opportunity for growth, however, it can become one.

Everything I have been through has gifted me with this "gift" and becoming an empath so that I can "see" the subtleties and help them grow. As mentors, we need to be better at planting the seed to cultivate the leaders of tomorrow. They may not always like what I say, because no one wants their weak parts on display. But it is essential for growth. Especially in medicine. Our patients deserve the best of us, and the only way through is by facing and accepting the dark.

Little did I know that I faced the dark to bring them to light so they could be the ripple in the pond. Through the embers, spreading like wildfire.

Looking back on my professional growth, I am amazed. I am proud. Hustling through all my training—both professionally and personally—despite failures, and restarting multiple times has really strengthened my foundation, providing the solid framework of my career focused on education. My younger self is so proud. Truthfully, I am not even sure I have grasped the significance of what I've accomplished. Especially since I have had such imposter syndrome around education, given dropping out of high school, earning a GED, to drop out again in college the first time because I was intimidated. I am truly in awe of how far I have come. It was the plan the whole time. God, the universe, spirit, however you relate, really does have a divine plan. Never did I ever think... Let alone being a mentor. It is fitting, given all I have been through.

I have been in a lot of leadership positions, completing my bachelor's degree, pursuing my master's as a PA, and full circle for the doctorate. I was on the board of directors for the Florida Academy of PAs, which would be equivalent to the Florida Medical Association (FMA), for seven consecutive years. I served in the House of Delegates and as an alternate delegate for the American Academy of PAs (AAPA), which would be equivalent to the American Medical Association (AMA). I have given local and national lectures on a variety of topics, from bullying, motivation, to case presentations. I have advocated for PAs on a state and national level, gone to local middle and high schools, been a part of a legacy leadership series for the American Chemical Society, volunteered for domestic violence, organized relief drives, and have won multiple awards for the hospital enterprise and for the state for my philanthropic efforts and mentoring. In addition to my PA and NP students, I mentor about 190 aspiring PAs (yes, I know every single one to detail), watching them grow and guiding them through their journey is heartwarming and my "why."

I've been featured on professional websites for all of the academic, clinical, and leadership roles that I've held. Currently, I am the program director and chair of the APP education committee, Grand Rounds within my organization. I'm confident I am leaving many things out, and even listing it here, I sometimes still don't believe it.

CATCHING FIRE

For those reading this, the pain, power gained, and recognition of purpose were worth it. Every heartache, disappointment, delay, even when it seemed to be treading quicksand. It is for a greater purpose. Yes, some have a harder path. Some have to overcome so much adversity, challenges, and completely break down to be rebuilt. When darkness falls upon you, there is a light. There always is. One cannot be without the other. The hardest part is not overcoming, but recognition and seeing the light in the darkness. Everyone has a rock, someone you can trust to stabilize you until you gain your footing. Some, however, are there for a moment. Others, for a lifetime. They *are* around you; you just have to be open to see them. To trust in something that you may not be able to "see" or understand at the moment. In the chaos, pause, step back, and look at what is happening. Breathe. Be open to possibilities, no matter what.

Each chapter, each version of me, I have been fortunate to have one person along this journey who has kept me focused, driven, and even protected. Yes, protection. Every single phase of my life, I have been bullied and challenged, and there have been multiple people throughout my life who have literally tried to "bring me down," trying to destroy me and all that I have worked for. Why? Well, I'm sure there are a lot of reasons. One thing for sure is that I know I hold a mirror to some. When they face the mirror, they don't like the reflection they see. While it is always in their control to change their circumstances, many do not have the stamina to do so. Many do not want to face their own demons. That is why many stay where they are. They are comfortable and do not want to grow. That requires change. That change includes facing all of yourself, even the demons, too, and *truly* coming to peace with every aspect of you. The good and bad. Yin and Yang. If you are reading this, you are here for a reason. You have the strength and ability. You just needed the little push, the validation that you are on the right path, and you can overcome all challenges laid before you.

People may not like you. That is okay. You may have very few friends, and that too is okay. One thing I have learned through all the challenges is that I do not need outside validation, and neither do you. Things, people, and circumstances will change. The only validation you need is from yourself. When you look in the mirror, love the reflection staring back. I look nothing like what I have been through, and the haters and the bullies don't like that. What

I love is they can't read me and every time I am knocked down, I come up stronger, more beautiful inside and out, and more determined to pay all the gratitude forward. The path is not easy. Nor should it be. It took a long time to get here, becoming the woman I have, and all the darkness I have faced would have broken them in a second. They would never have survived. How do I know? Because their character is showing. For someone to behave as they do, they are unhappy, unhealed, and stuck in their misery.

My power is mine. I have earned all I have gone through and chose to take "The Road Less Travelled," in the words of Robert Frost. I will continue to be a voice for what's right and just. They will never take my power from me. Everything I have been through has molded me into a strong, resilient, intelligent, compassionate woman whose only wish is to guide others to their best selves. I do not lose sleep over any of these individuals who have tried any more. While it is annoying and can be incredibly frustrating, even to the point of questioning things, I am actually thankful for them. I do not harbor resentment or any ill will. I do not want that negative energy. I have spent my entire life strengthening my self-esteem, confidence, and self-love. Giving my power away to them is not worth the cost. I have learned to alchemize it. So, with each attack, I will level up. I will use the energy they put out to continue to become the ripple in the pond, helping others. The haters hate that. They can plot and scheme. But me? I'll keep building. I'll keep moving forward, focused on a peaceful, happy future and leaving a legacy behind.

I am incredibly thankful for each of my mentors. Each person who has put up with, strengthened, and fostered my growth. You know who you are, and I am blessed to have you. Each of you holds a very special place in my heart. This book is not just a reflection and a diary of my own growth, but a celebration of your hard work as well. Words could never express the gratitude I have for you.

CHAPTER 16

THE RISE OF THE PHOENIX

I do think about *what's next.* I know that I love clinical medicine. I'm good at it, but I love teaching, mentoring, and motivating too. I am not sure what the universe has in store for me next. At the current time, I am grateful for it all. I have no regrets in life. I would do everything the same if offered the opportunity to go back in time. Everything I've done, all I have healed, has prepared me for this beautiful life I have. It's led me here. Writing this book, being a voice for the voiceless and the lighthouse.

Being of service, being of use, is the most rewarding thing I can think of doing, with boundaries. I wouldn't have it any other way. The medical field, in many ways, saved me from myself. Now, I try to pay it forward to others as much as possible. Teaching, guiding others how to use the pain for good and realizing that everything, everyone has a purpose. The light is always there. A quote from online, not really sure who wrote it, but "the cracks are where the light enters."

We must break to rebuild. Each rebuild brings us one step closer to our purpose. None of us is promised tomorrow, so if you want to make changes, the time is never going to be right. Just do it. Begin now. Do it scared. Do it broke. Just do it. The saying that we are not defined by what has happened to us but by how we react couldn't be truer. As a young, timid woman, untrusting of my own abilities, I grew into a strong, compassionate, capable, intelligent woman, and I sit here reflecting—and it feels so surreal. It's as if I've lived many lifetimes. Each chapter broken down to ash, only to rise stronger and more resilient than before. With the turn of each page, we are anew, embracing the challenges of the past as we forge a way forward, creating a life we love. With a sense of purpose and understanding, we are never alone and truly are capable of everything we set our hearts to. There's another saying. I don't know who said it, but it goes, if you keep your face to the sunshine, you'll never see the darkness. Who the hell wants a life like that? You need the darkness to see the light. You can't appreciate the light without having experienced the dark. That's the purpose of this book: to show you that you can be Dark Phoenix for a quarter of your life or more. All kinds of things that are done to you, but we must recognize that some are because we carry others' burdens and choose to live as victims, which is a lot of what I've done. Isolation, and especially after my parents' divorce, I did a lot of that to myself because I felt unworthy. For some reason that I concocted, because my biological parents didn't want me, I was defective. As I've gotten older, I realize the stronger sense of love that was so hard to realize is that I was actually chosen by two people who didn't even *want* children, but both wanted *me*. That, to me, is something special, and it took a long time to see *that it* is love, regardless of if they knew how to show it in the way that I *expected* it to be shown. They did the best with what they had and by what they knew at that time.

I'm not overly religious; my mom is not either. We are more spiritual than religious. But she says that the universe or God had made a mistake and ultimately corrected it by placing me with her and Steven. I could have taken my life as the victim, played that role, and become nothing. I could have used that as my crutch my whole life, or an excuse. I chose to live a full life with a sense of purpose. The choice is yours.

Mentoring, teaching, healing, and my two big projects will hopefully come to fruition soon, and I will know that I have left my mark on the hospital, the people who work there, and those who come for help there in a truly impactful way. I'm not sure what could be more wonderful as a legacy than that. So, my advice: time is going by anyway. Make the best of the moments and always choose to invest in yourself. I am grateful for every single person who has pushed me along the way. Especially those who tried to bring me down. You, most of all, fueled my growth. Igniting my passion, allowing those embers to spread, and strengthening my purpose…

The Rise of The Phoenix.

ACKNOWLEDGMENTS

Mom - thank you for giving me a second chance at life. Thank you for loving me sight unseen and for choosing me. I love you — forever and unconditionally, in every lifetime.

Sam - you are my heart and my best friend. Life is both beautiful and cruel, and you possess the rare gift of seeing the good in it despite everything. That light within you makes the lives of those around you better. You make this world better.

The ro-aaaad ahead may be uncertain, but I have unwavering confidence in you and your ability to overcome every challenge. You deserve — and are worthy of — everything life has to offer.

I love you. Forever and unconditionally.

To the unknown individual and their family who heard a baby crying in a home for days and chose to call the authorities - You are the catalyst for all of this. Words could never fully express how blessed I am that you were there. You are a hero to me. You saved my life.

Thank you.

To my family, mentors, friends, colleagues, professors, and even the strangers I have had the honor of knowing — From the bottom of my heart, thank you.

When I was lost, confused, or broken, you saw me — even when I could not see myself. You know who you are. Everything I am is, in part, because of you. I would not be here — let alone writing this book — if your light had not pierced the darkness.

Each of you helped guide me back home to myself — stronger, resilient, compassionate — so that I may now be a lighthouse for others.

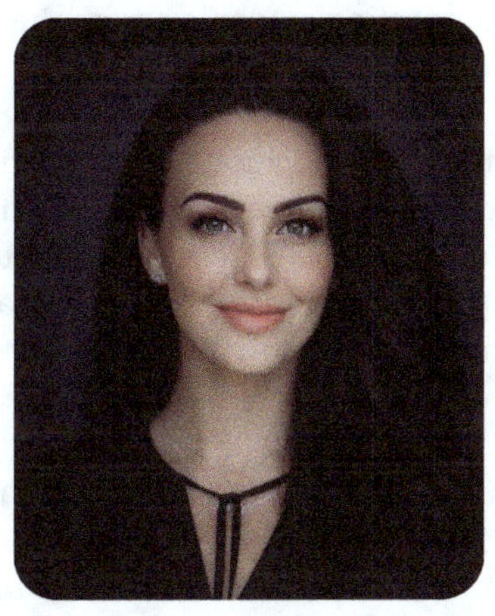

Dr. Nicole Schtupak, DMSc, PA-C, RDMS, is a nationally recognized medical professional, educator, researcher, and advocate whose life and career are defined by resilience, leadership, and service.

Abandoned as an infant and left fighting for her life, she transformed unimaginable beginnings into a distinguished healthcare career spanning more than 25 years. A multi-specialty Physician Associate (PA) with experience in infectious disease, emergency medicine, critical care, internal medicine, and interventional radiology, she also brings over two decades of experience as a multi-credentialed Registered Diagnostic Medical Sonographer, with research contributions in genetics and thyroid cancer.

For more than 20 years, Dr. Schtupak has served at Cleveland Clinic Weston, where she currently leads as Program Director and Chair of the APP Education Committee. A passionate mentor, she has guided hundreds of pre-medical, nursing, aspiring, and current PA students and has dedicated her career to strengthening clinical education nationwide. During the COVID-19 pandemic, she played a pivotal role in connecting students across the country with preceptors to prevent disruptions in their training.

Her academic contributions include the publication of a rare infective endocarditis case—one of only twenty-seven reported globally and the seventh documented instance in the United States, causing disease in a prosthetic aortic valve—demonstrating her commitment to advancing clinical knowledge and excellence in patient care.

Dr. Schtupak has served seven consecutive years on the Florida Academy of PAs Board of Directors, including as Vice President and South Regional Director, and was elected to the AAPA House of Delegates as Delegate and Delegate-Elect. Her leadership and advocacy efforts have earned multiple professional honors and national recognition.

Beyond medicine, she is deeply committed to community engagement, organizing relief drives, healthcare outreach initiatives, domestic violence awareness efforts, and educational programs that empower patients to take ownership of their health.

Through her writing and speaking, she champions resilience, purpose-driven leadership, and the belief that our beginnings do not determine our destiny.

When she is not working or mentoring, she finds peace in gardening, stargazing, beach sunsets, and dreaming of autumn mountains despite being a Florida native.

www.ingramcontent.com/pod-product-compliance
Lightning Source LLC
Chambersburg PA
CBHW061528050726
47593CB00002B/714